THE
COMPLETE
BOOK OF
MASSAGE

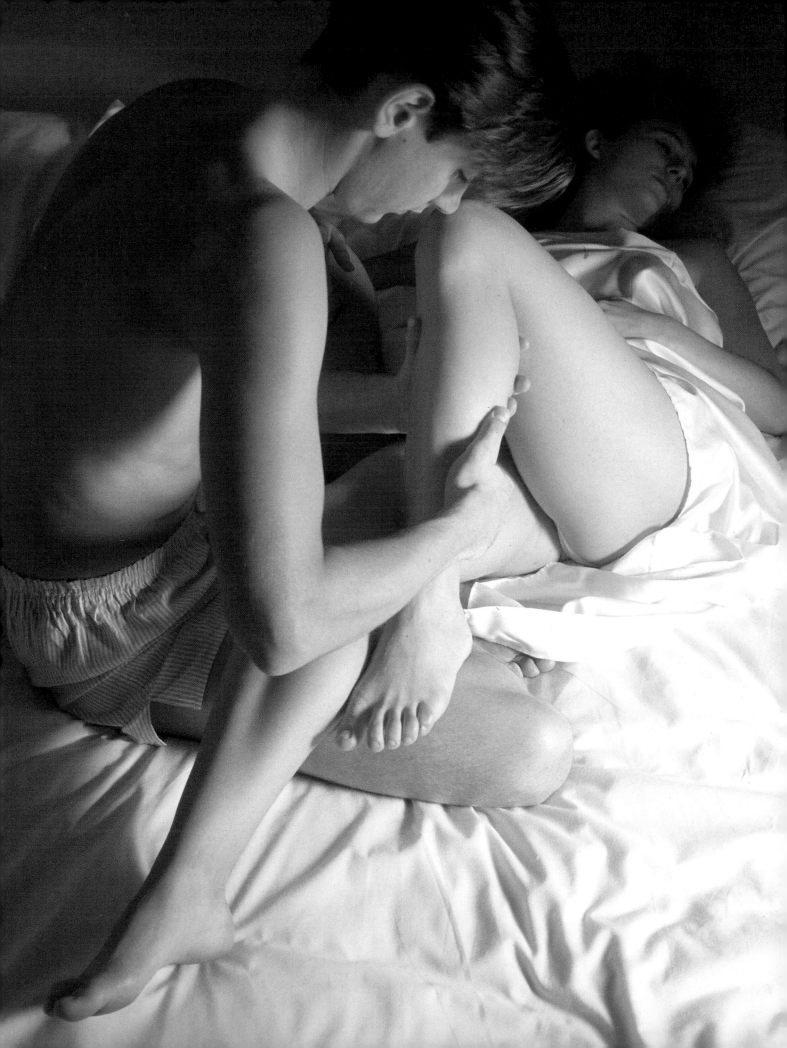

THE
COMPLETE
BOOK OF
MASSAGE

·

CLARE
MAXWELL-
HUDSON

Photography by Sandra Lousada

DORLING KINDERSLEY · LONDON

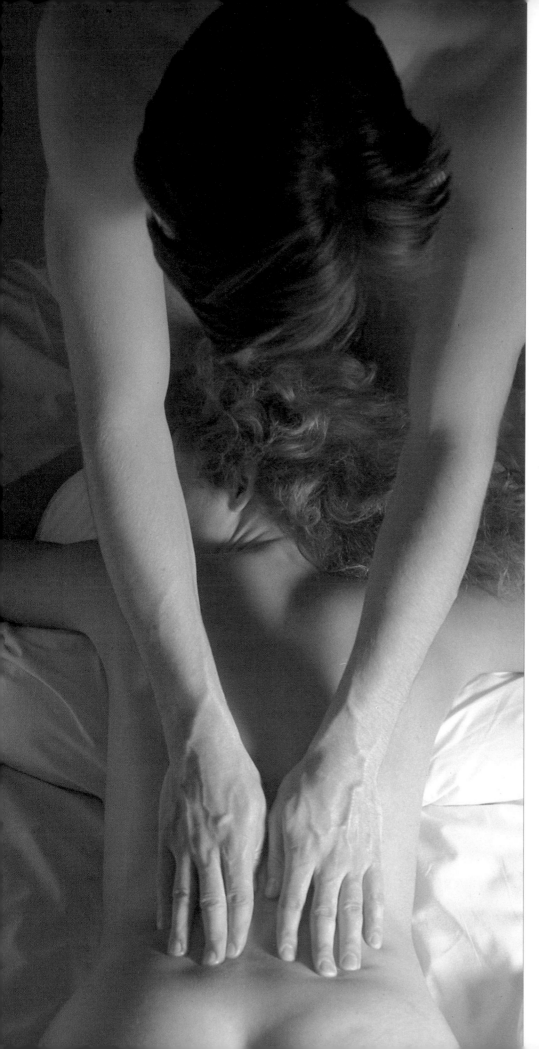

To Miles,
with thanks for all your help

EDITOR *Claire Le Bas*
ART EDITOR *Mark Richards*

ART DIRECTOR *Anne-Marie Bulat*
MANAGING EDITOR *Daphne Razazan*

First published in Great Britain in 1988
by Dorling Kindersley Publishers Limited,
9 Henrietta Street, London, WC2E 8PS.

Reprinted 1993

BRITISH LIBRARY
CATALOGUING IN PUBLICATION DATA

Maxwell-Hudson, Clare
    Massage, the Complete Book of
    1. Massage
    I. Title
    615.8'22   RM721

    ISBN 0-86318-290-9
    ISBN 0-86318-281-X   Pbk

Printed and bound in Italy
by Arnoldo Mondadori Editore, Verona

CONTENTS

1

Giving a Massage

2

Self-Massage

3

Babies and Children

4

Pressure Techniques

5

Therapeutic Massage

INTRODUCTION

Massage is one of the easiest ways of attaining and maintaining good health and something we all do naturally. It is a healing instinct, innate in us all, to rub an aching shoulder or stroke a furrowed brow. Headaches, aches and pains, insomnia, tension and stress can all be alleviated with one simple instrument – our hands.

The basis of massage is touch, and there is increasing medical evidence to show the great value of touch. In a research project at Harvard Medical School a number of patients all about to undergo similar operations were divided into two groups. The anaesthetist visited all the patients the night before the operation. To one group he gave the usual information about the procedure for the following day. He gave similar information to the other group, but spent about five minutes longer with each patient; he sat on their beds, held their hands and was generally warm and sympathetic. After the operation, patients who had received the friendly approach asked for only about half the quantity of drugs that the others requested, and on average were discharged from hospital three days earlier. This suggests the powerful effect that friendliness, combined with warmth, sympathy and touch, can have on general health.

Touch is so natural to us that without it people can become depressed and irritable. Observations show that children brought up in families where parents and children touch each other are healthier and more able to withstand pain and infection than children deprived of touch. They sleep better, are more sociable and generally happier.

But our need for touch does not stop at childhood, we all need it to give us a feeling of love, warmth and security. In fact, the Marriage Guidance Council advises couples to touch each other more. It goes as far as to say that the rising rate of divorce could be due to lack of physical contact within families. Perhaps just a few minutes spent massaging each other could prevent numerous ills, physical and mental.

SOCIAL INHIBITIONS

Despite all this evidence to show the benefits of touch, we are still hesitant about touching each other. I think this is due to a confusion between sensuality and sexuality. Because we are so afraid of the connection between sex and touch, we have formalized touch. There are only a few occasions when adults are allowed to touch each other freely. Massage removes the taboos of touching and allows people to touch in a positive way.

OUR DESIRE TO TOUCH

Not feeling free to touch each other, we turn to our children or our pets. It is natural for mothers to cuddle and rock their babies. Friends and

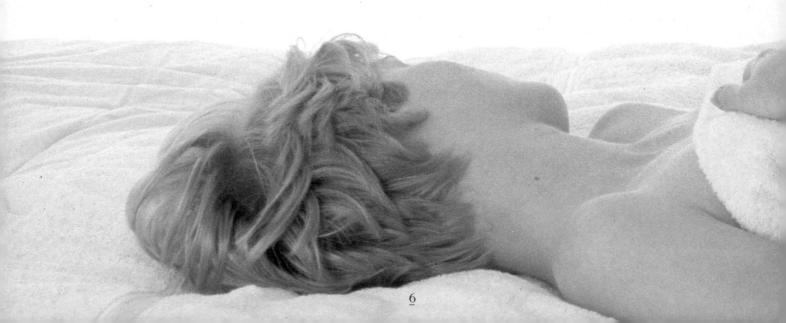

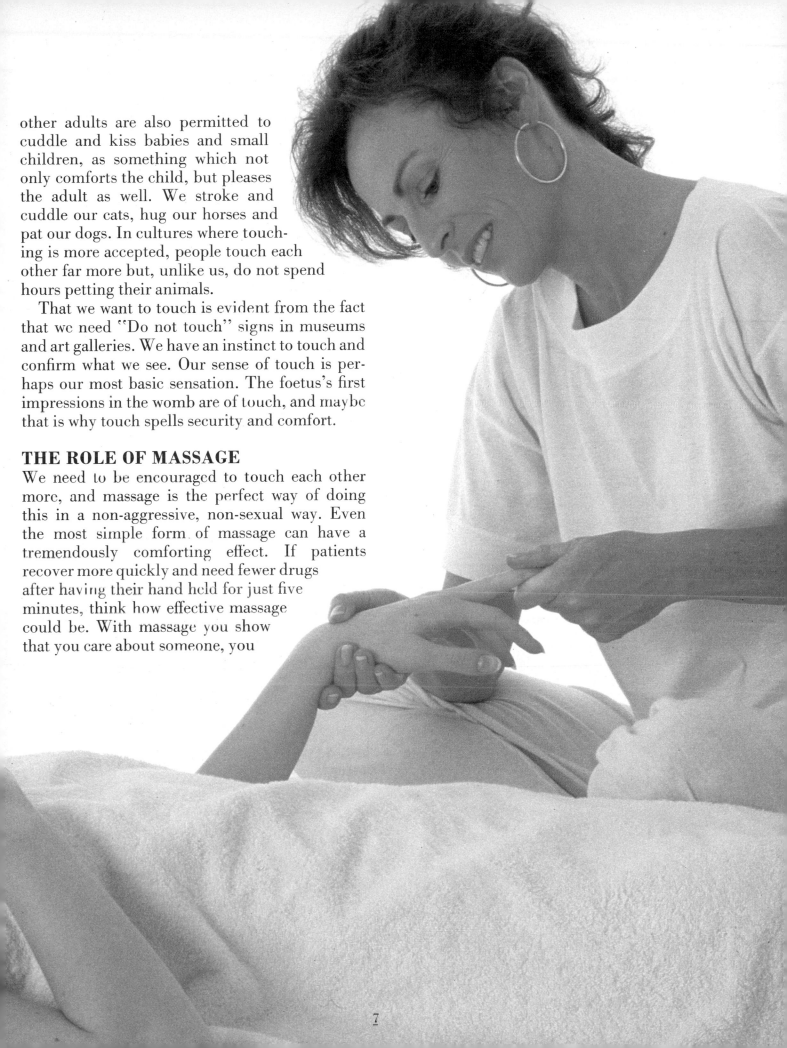

other adults are also permitted to cuddle and kiss babies and small children, as something which not only comforts the child, but pleases the adult as well. We stroke and cuddle our cats, hug our horses and pat our dogs. In cultures where touching is more accepted, people touch each other far more but, unlike us, do not spend hours petting their animals.

That we want to touch is evident from the fact that we need "Do not touch" signs in museums and art galleries. We have an instinct to touch and confirm what we see. Our sense of touch is perhaps our most basic sensation. The foetus's first impressions in the womb are of touch, and maybe that is why touch spells security and comfort.

THE ROLE OF MASSAGE

We need to be encouraged to touch each other more, and massage is the perfect way of doing this in a non-aggressive, non-sexual way. Even the most simple form of massage can have a tremendously comforting effect. If patients recover more quickly and need fewer drugs after having their hand held for just five minutes, think how effective massage could be. With massage you show that you care about someone, you convey a sense of sharing and intuitive understanding, reassurance and pleasure.

BENEFITS OF MASSAGE

Massage has profound effects on the health of the person being massaged. It improves circulation, relaxes muscles, aids digestion and, by stimulating the lymphatic system, it speeds up the elimination of waste products. These direct benefits, combined with the psychological benefits of feeling cared for and cosseted, quickly produce a marvellous feeling of well-being that cannot be matched by modern drugs.

The benefits of massage are felt not only by the person being massaged: the masseur benefits just as much. Some interesting observations back this up: it has been discovered that when stroking a pet we soothe ourselves too, and our blood pressure goes down. I maintain that giving a massage produces the same effect – stroking a person has the same relaxing quality for both the giver and receiver.

ACTIVE MEDITATION

To me, giving a massage is like active meditation. In order to give a good massage, you should be calm and completely absorbed in what you are doing. Concentrating on the rhythm of your massage, you will soon relax totally, and your relaxation will be transmitted to the person you are massaging. When you massage in this state, you will find that you not only give a better massage, but that when you finish you are full of energy, refreshed and revitalized. Even if you start giving a massage feeling irritated, anxious or upset, you will find that it is virtually impossible to remain in a bad mood while doing the soothing, hypnotic massage strokes.

HISTORY OF MASSAGE

Massage probably goes as far back in history as the existence of man. It is something that we all do instinctively: apes grooming each other, animals licking their wounds and men rubbing an aching joint are all using massage. It is probably the oldest form of medical treatment, and has been used throughout history by all cultures.

It was called anatripsis by the Greek physician, Hippocrates, and referred to as tripsis, friction, manipulation, rubbing or shampooing by other writers. Our use of the word massage is relatively new, and probably derives from the Arabic word "masah", which means to stroke with the hand.

Ancient Chinese, Indian and Egyptian manuscripts refer to the use of massage to prevent and cure diseases and to heal injuries. The earliest mention of massage appears in a Chinese book dating from about 2700 BC: "Early morning stroking with the palm of the hand, after the night's sleep, when the blood is rested and the tempers relaxed, protects against colds, keeps the organs supple and prevents minor ailments."

In ancient Greek and Roman literature there are numerous references to massage. It was advocated before and after sport, instead of exercise during convalescence, after bathing or as a medical treatment for such varied conditions as melancholia, asthma, digestive problems and even sterility.

The Roman emperor's physician, Galen (131-210 AD), wrote at least 16 books relating to massage and exercise, and many of his ideas are still relevant today. He classified massage into firm, gentle and moderate, and wrote "I direct that the strokes and circuits of the hands should be made of many sorts, in order that as far as possible all the muscle fibres should be rubbed in every direction." He describes massage given to the gladiators before and after the games: "They were anointed with oil and rubbed until they were red." Julius Caesar was massaged daily to relieve neuralgia; the Roman writer Pliny was so indebted to his foreign masseur that he requested the emperor to grant him the highest honour, Roman citizenship.

Massage has always been greatly valued in India, and practically everyone you meet there knows how to massage. Mothers massage their babies, and later these children are taught to do the same for their parents. Massage is incorporated in Ayurvedic treatments – an Indian system of medicine dating back to 1800 BC – with herbs, spices and aromatic oils being rubbed into the skin.

Other cultures, too, have always relied on massage to maintain health. In Sir George Simpson's record of his travels, "Voyage around the World" (1889), he writes of the Sandwich Islanders: "He or she fares sumptuously every day, or rather, every hour, and takes little or no exercise, while the constant habit of being shampooed (massaged) after every meal, and oftener if desirable or expedient, promotes circulation or digestion without superinducing either exhaustion or fatigue." Captain Cook recorded how, in 1779, his painful sciatica was cured when twelve women from Tahiti massaged him from head to foot.

In the 18th and 19th centuries, massage grew in popularity in Europe, under the influence of a Swede, Per Henrik Ling (1776-1839), whose system of Swedish massage spread throughout Europe. He laid great emphasis on medical gymnastics and massage, and classified his treatments as passive or gymnastic movements, pressure, friction, vibration, percussion or rotation. His work was rewarded by the Crown, an institute was set up in Stockholm, and in 1838 a Swedish Institute was opened in London. By the turn of the century, such institutes could be found in Russia, France and America. Ling's influence has lasted, and massage is still frequently referred to as Swedish massage.

At the end of the 19th century, massage was a popular medical treatment, and was frequently used by eminent surgeons, cardiologists and physicians, who either performed the massage themselves or trained people (usually women) to do it for them. But "houses of ill fame" also used the word "massage" as a cloak for their activities, and so in London in 1894 eight professional women banded together to form the Society of Trained Masseurs. They were the founders of what is now known as the Chartered Society of Physiotherapy.

During the First World War, massage was used extensively in the treatment of nerve injury and shell-shock. However, the use of electrical apparatus became increasingly fashionable and, in the UK, hand massage was relegated to a back seat. Its use was considered pampering rather than therapeutic. It was believed that equally good results could be obtained with modern drugs or machinery, but experience has shown that drugs have side-effects and nothing can replace the human hand.

Today once again, the therapeutic value of massage is being recognized. It is regaining its rightful place in health care, as a complement to other medical treatments, and as a means of helping us all to maintain positive health.

THE MAGIC OF MASSAGE

This old oriental tale demonstrates the power of massage.

Once upon a time there was a young woman called Fatima, who was constantly scolded and nagged by her mother-in-law. Eventually Fatima could no longer stand this, and went to the local herbalist for some poison to kill the old woman. After some thought, the herbalist gave her a heavily scented potion. He told her that this should be massaged into the skin daily, and that after six weeks her mother-in-law would die.

Fatima did as she was instructed, and each day she gave her mother-in-law a massage. Gradually the old woman's vicious temper seemed to disappear, an empathy grew between the two women, and after a while they started to understand each other.

Fatima began to regret her desire to kill her mother-in-law, and as time ran out she became increasingly worried. Finally she returned to the herbalist and begged for an antidote to the poison. The wise old man smiled and explained that no antidote was needed. The poison she had been massaging into the old woman's skin was simply a mixture of aromatic oils — the antidote to her situation.

I hope that as it did for Fatima and her mother-in-law, massage will enhance your life.

Clare Maxwell-Hudson

CLARE MAXWELL-HUDSON

In order for a massage to have the maximum benefit, it is important that it is given in a comfortable environment. During the massage, your partner or friend should feel cosseted, so choose a warm, peaceful room with dim lights, where neither of you will be disturbed. Have plenty of towels available to cover him or her, so that only the area you are massaging is exposed – he won't relax properly if he is cold. In winter, a small electric pad or a hot water bottle under the back feels wonderful.

Massage surface

Your friend should lie on a firm, padded surface. I like to massage on the floor for several reasons: everyone can find enough space on the floor, so there is no excuse not to massage, and you can practise anywhere at any time. I also like the fact that the person being massaged can spread out and that there is plenty of space around me. Pad the floor with a piece of foam rubber or a couple of thick blankets, and kneel on something soft, to avoid sore, calloused knees. Use cushions and rolled up towels to make your friend comfortable.

If you suffer from painful knees or a bad back, you will probably find it easier to work at a table. A large kitchen table is ideal: it should reach about the top of your thighs, and it must be sturdy enough to hold the weight of your friend and your weight as you lean into the massage. Again, pad the surface with a piece of foam rubber or some blankets.

If you do not have a suitable table, you can buy a portable massage couch. They are about 6 feet long and 2 feet wide (2m × 60cm), and roughly the height of a normal table.

Most beds are too soft for a massage – all the pressure is absorbed by the mattress – and they are often an awkward height for giving a massage. However, if you want to give a soothing, soporific massage, a bed may be ideal because you can leave your friend asleep when you finish.

YOUR COMFORT

You need to be relaxed to give a good massage, so your own comfort is extremely important. With practice, you will learn to work without tensing your own muscles. Massage should be as relaxing to give as it is to receive.

Your posture

Keep your back straight throughout the massage, and use the weight of your body to give both rhythm and depth to your massage. If you are working at a table, keep your feet wide apart and bend your knees so that you can lean into the strokes. If you are working on the floor, kneel with your knees apart or, if you find it more comfortable, have one knee on the floor and the other one up with that foot on the floor. Never stay in one position for long; always face in the direction of your massage strokes – face the head when working up the body, and face across the body when working across.

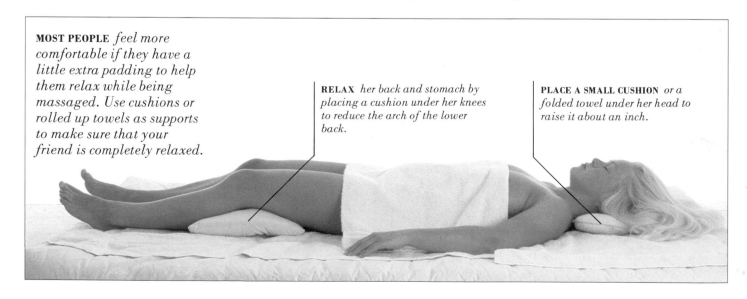

MOST PEOPLE *feel more comfortable if they have a little extra padding to help them relax while being massaged. Use cushions or rolled up towels as supports to make sure that your friend is completely relaxed.*

RELAX *her back and stomach by placing a cushion under her knees to reduce the arch of the lower back.*

PLACE A SMALL CUSHION *or a folded towel under her head to raise it about an inch.*

Your clothes

Wear loose-fitting, washable clothes and flat shoes or go barefoot. Remove all jewellery before you give a massage: rings can scratch the skin, and bracelets or necklaces can jangle or trail over it, which is distracting and irritating.

Exercising your hands

Your hands are your tools, so it is worth exercising them to increase their sensitivity and flexibility (see right for exercises to keep your hands supple). To heighten their sensitivity, hold them close together without letting them touch. Draw them about 5cm (2in) apart, then back until they are almost touching. Now take them 10cm (4in) apart, then return them to their original position. Continue like this, expanding the gap gradually until your hands are about 25cm (10in) apart, then bring them very slowly together. You will probably experience an unusual sensation, perhaps heat or tingling, or a pulsating or magnetic sensation.

GUIDELINES

You can tailor a massage to suit any needs; even a single technique can be stimulating or soothing, depending on how you do it. A firm, brisk massage is invigorating, while slow, steady strokes can send someone to sleep. The fun of massage is experimenting. You never need to do the same massage twice – each time you massage, find out your friend's needs, and give a massage

KEEPING YOUR HANDS SUPPLE

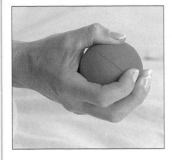

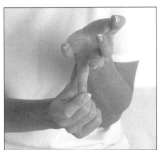

1 Hold a small rubber ball in one hand and repeatedly squeeze and relax your fingers round it. Then repeat with the other hand.

2 Rotate and stretch each finger and thumb in turn. Grasp one finger with your other hand, rotate it in each direction, then pull it gently.

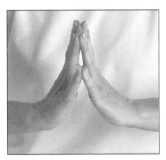

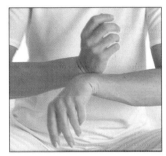

3 Put your hands together, then lift your elbows up so that your palms no longer touch. Press your fingers against each other, and hold for six seconds.

4 Put the inside of one wrist on the back of the other, with your elbows out. Roll your hands round each other, making as large a circle as possible.

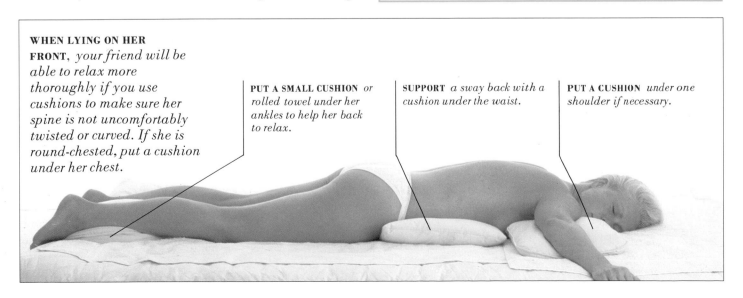

WHEN LYING ON HER FRONT, *your friend will be able to relax more thoroughly if you use cushions to make sure her spine is not uncomfortably twisted or curved. If she is round-chested, put a cushion under her chest.*

PUT A SMALL CUSHION *or rolled towel under her ankles to help her back to relax.*

SUPPORT *a sway back with a cushion under the waist.*

PUT A CUSHION *under one shoulder if necessary.*

to suit them. Whether you follow a sequence rigorously or improvise your own techniques, the following tips will help make your massage a wonderful experience.

■ The most important element of a massage is rhythm. A rhythmic massage will send waves of relaxation through the body.

■ Massage should be pleasurable, so ask your friend to tell you if anything you do is unpleasant or painful.

■ Mould your hands to the contours of the body, and imagine you are sculpting the body into its perfect shape.

■ Keep one hand in contact with the body throughout the massage of any area. Ideally, your whole body massage should feel like one continuous, flowing stroke.

■ Vary your pressure from very light to very strong. It should be lighter over bony areas and firmer over large muscles. Don't be afraid to apply deep pressure: a firm touch feels good.

■ It is never necessary to use force during your massage, simply use the weight of your body to apply pressure.

■ Concentrate on the massage, and do not talk much. Your massage will be more effective if both of you focus attention on the various sensations.

■ Do not worry if your first movements seem clumsy. All touch feels good, and with practice your massage will become flowing and confident.

■ You will find it easier to learn with a partner or friend rather than by yourself, because you can try the techniques out on each other and see how they should feel.

■ To give a good massage you need to be totally relaxed, so don't try too hard. If in doubt about what to do next, just stroke. As long as your movements are rhythmic, the massage will feel interesting and relaxing.

Dealing with tension

Any areas that feel stiff, taut or lumpy need extra massage to dispel tension. Small lumps under the skin are caused by bunched-up muscle fibres or an accumulation of waste products. Ease out the tension by applying pressure directly on the area or by stroking the surrounding area. Don't press

---

A WORD OF WARNING

Though massage is of enormous benefit, there are some occasions when you should not massage. Never massage someone with any of the following conditions unless his doctor gives permission.

■ An infection, a contagious disease or a high temperature.

■ Acute back pain, especially if the pain shoots down the arms or legs when you massage the back.

■ A skin infection, bruising or acute inflammation.

■ An inflammatory condition such as thrombosis or phlebitis.

See pages 126 to 137 for more information on massaging people in ill-health.

---

too hard: if you hurt someone, his muscles will automatically tense up, destroying the work you have already done. Don't spend too long on the area, but keep returning to it until it is relaxed.

Ticklishness

An area of ticklishness is usually caused by nervous tension. Slightly increase the pressure of your massage and persevere in that area. If this does not help, move on to the surrounding area. When this is relaxed, return to the original area and it will probably no longer be ticklish.

MASSAGE SEQUENCE

There is no single correct sequence for giving a massage, it depends on your and your friend's preferences. I always teach the back massage first: it is a large area, and most of the massage techniques are used on it. Almost everyone loves having their back massaged, so you will get favourable comments when you first start, which is encouraging.

When I give a professional body massage, I usually start with the back or the feet. Again, most people enjoy having their feet massaged, and you can relax the whole body with a foot massage. It also means that if you are going to talk (and you easily might at the beginning of a massage), you can look at each other as you speak. This is particularly important with people who are slightly nervous, because they can gain confidence in you by watching you.

My massage usually follows the sequence below, but you can vary it as much as you like.
1 Right foot and leg, left foot and leg
2 Left hand and arm, right hand and arm
3 Abdomen
4 Back of legs, back
5 Chest, face and head.

Timing

A whole body massage usually takes about an hour, or 1½ hours if you include the face and head. If you have only limited time, concentrate on just two or three areas rather than rush through a whole massage. I find that the quickest way to relax someone is to massage the shoulders, face and head.

Aromatic oils

Your massage will be greatly enhanced if you use oil to help your hands glide over the skin. Some people use talcum powder as a lubricant, but I find that my hands move more freely with oil.

Use a light vegetable oil either on its own or scented with essential oils (see Aromatherapy, pages 18 to 20). Keep your oil in a plastic bottle with a narrow opening so that it is easy to add a few drops of oil during the massage, and so that you don't spill much if you knock the bottle over. Keep an open bottle of oil within easy reach throughout the massage.

BREATHING

When concentrating on something new, people often become tense and forget to breathe. Breathe deeply and slowly, and try to stay as relaxed as possible. Don't try too hard – the more relaxed you are, the better your massage will be.

Proper breathing is fundamental to our health and ability to relax. Many people breathe incorrectly, which can lead to a variety of health problems, including angina, insomnia, anxiety, dizziness and tingling in the hands and feet.

Check whether you breathe properly: put one hand on your chest and the other on your stomach, and breathe normally. Which hand moves? It should be the one on your stomach. A great many of us breathe from the chest, taking short, shallow breaths rather than long, deep ones. This is part of the normal response to stress, and over long periods it upsets the delicate balance of oxygen and carbon dioxide in the body.

Breathing correctly makes you feel calmer, and will prevent you becoming tense while you give a massage, so it is worth practising. Sit or lie comfortably and put your hands on your abdomen. Breathe in for a count of three and feel your abdomen expand. Then breathe out for a count of four, and feel your abdomen fall.

When you give a massage, you can teach your friend how to breathe correctly. Put one hand on his chest and the other on his abdomen. As he breathes out, press gently down on the abdomen, and release the pressure when he breathes in.

USING THE OIL
Never pour the oil directly onto the body. Pour about a teaspoon of oil into the palm of one hand, rub your hands together to warm it slightly, then stroke the oil onto the body. During the massage, one hand should always remain in contact with the body, so whenever you need to add a little more oil, follow the sequence shown.

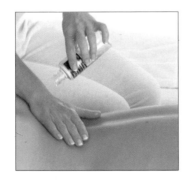

1 Pour a little oil onto the back of one hand, still stroking slowly with this hand as you do so.

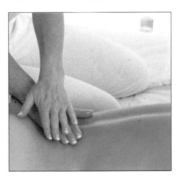

2 Continue stroking and place your free hand lightly on top of the massaging hand.

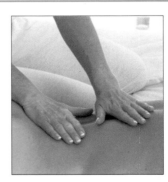

3 Stroke the oil onto the body from the back of your hand, and continue your massage.

BASIC TECHNIQUES

The wonderful thing about massage is that it is very easy. Once you have mastered a few basic movements, you can give a complete body massage. Most other techniques used in a massage are simply variations on the movements shown here. Practise on the back to start with.

STROKING

The rhythmic, flowing movements of stroking form the basis of a massage, and they are the ones you will use most. Use them to apply the oil and to link other movements. If ever you can't think what to do next in your massage, just stroke. You can do a whole body massage using only stroking movements, giving variety and interest simply by changing the speed and pressure of the strokes. Slow movements are calming, while brisk movements are stimulating. Stroking improves the circulation, relaxes tense muscles and soothes jangled nerves. With this most basic of all massage movements, the secret is to be utterly relaxed yourself so that the movements just flow.

FAN STROKING

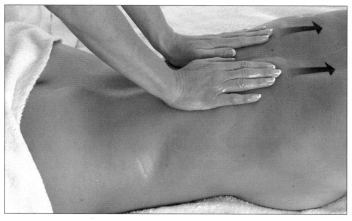

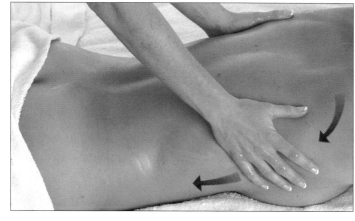

1 This is the simplest type of stroking and is used on almost all areas of the body. Start with your hands side by side and glide them slowly upwards, leading with your fingers. Lean onto your hands to apply a steady, even pressure through the palms and heels.

2 Fan your hands out, reducing pressure as you do so, and slide them down the sides. Mould your hands to the shape of the body so that your stroke covers the whole area: your friend will notice if any bits get left out. Stroke smoothly and gently, taking care not to drag the skin.

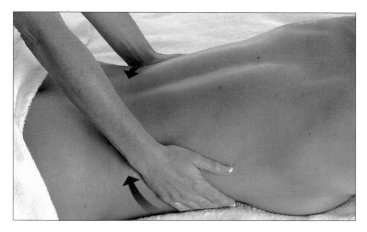

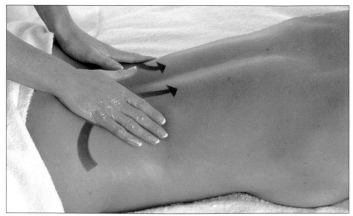

3 Pull your hands up the sides, keeping them relaxed and moulded to the curves of the body. When stroking the back or abdomen, squeeze in slightly at the waist as you pull your hands up. On other parts of the body, keep this return movement very light.

4 Applying hardly any pressure, swivel your hands round ready to start again. You can vary the length of the stroke, but always keep the whole movement smooth and continuous. As a general rule, stroke firmly towards the heart and glide lightly back down again.

CIRCLE STROKING

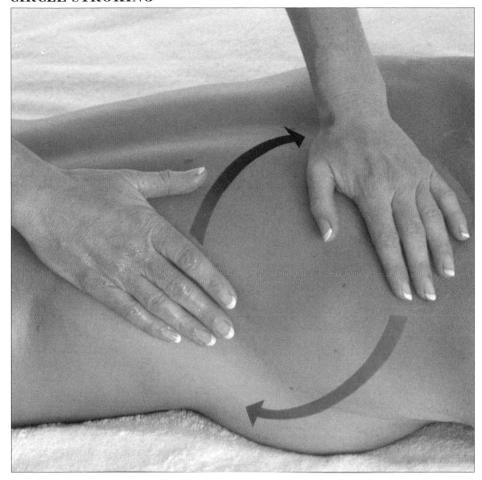

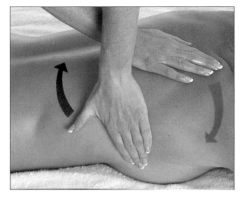

2 Your arms cross as one hand completes the circle. One hand does a whole circle while the other does only half a circle.

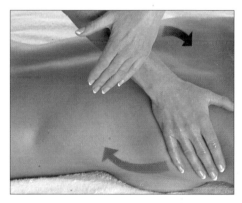

1 This continuous circling movement gives a lovely flowing sensation. Place both hands on one side of the body, about 15cm (6in)

apart, then stroke round in wide curves, making a circle. Press firmly on the upwards and outwards stroke, and gently as you glide down and in.

3 Lift one hand over the other arm, and continue stroking with the other hand. Place your hand gently on the skin and repeat.

CAT STROKING

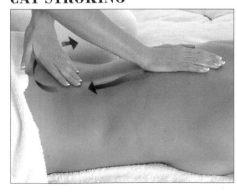

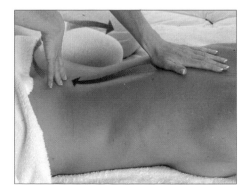

THUMB STROKING

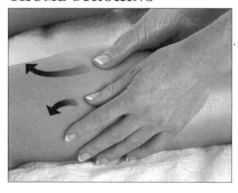

1 This is a very soothing, soporific movement. Stroke slowly down the body, one hand following the other. Apply virtually no pressure so that your hands barely touch the skin.

2 Lift the first hand off and return it through the air to start again. The return movement should be as smooth as the stroking, to make the whole stroke rhythmic and continuous.

On smaller areas, stroke with just your thumbs. Stroke firmly upwards and out to the side with one thumb. Follow with the other, stroking up a little higher and out the other side.

KNEADING

This movement is just like kneading dough, and is useful on the shoulders and fleshy areas such as the hips and thighs. It stretches and relaxes tense muscles, improves the circulation, bringing fresh blood and nutrients to the area, and helps the absorption and elimination of waste products. You can vary the effect by changing the depth and speed of kneading: slow and deep, or fast and stimulating. Light kneading affects the skin and top layer of muscles; firm kneading affects the deeper muscles. Use enough oil so that your hands move freely without sliding around uncontrollably.

BASIC KNEADING

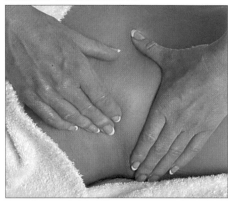

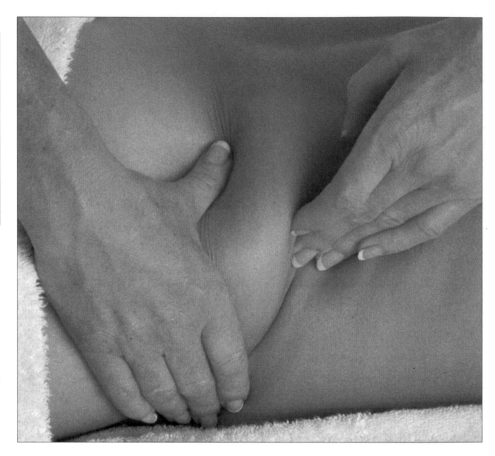

1 Place your hands flat on the skin with the fingers pointing away from you and your elbows out to the sides. Press down with the palm of one hand, then grasp the flesh between your fingers and thumb and push it towards the other hand.

2 ▶ Release the flesh and grasp it with the second hand. Rhythmically squeeze and release flesh with alternate hands, one hand releasing as the other compresses.

WRINGING▶

For a deeper and more stimulating movement, add a twist to the basic kneading. Imagine you are wringing out a towel: pull the flesh up with one hand and across towards your other hand, pressing deeply into it with the thumb of the other hand.

LIGHT KNEADING▶▶

On less fleshy areas, such as the shoulders and upper arms, knead more lightly. Lift, squeeze and roll the flesh between the thumb and fingers of one hand, glide it towards the other hand, and squeeze the flesh with the second hand.

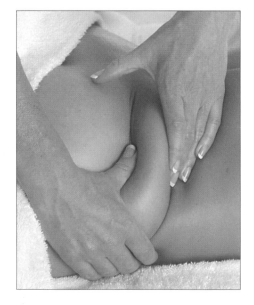

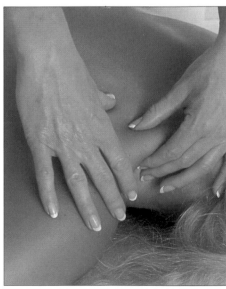

PRESSURES

Deep, direct pressure is extremely useful for releasing tension in the muscles on either side of the spine and around the shoulders, and is also very relaxing. Apply the pressure gradually and steadily, and never poke sharply. Use very little oil so that your hands do not slide around, and make sure that your thumb nails do not gouge the skin.

STATIC PRESSURE

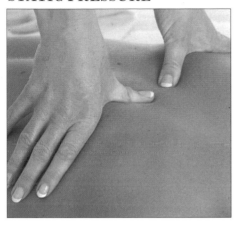

Place the pads of your thumbs on the skin and gradually lean onto them. Press for a few seconds, then release and glide to the next point.

CIRCULAR PRESSURE

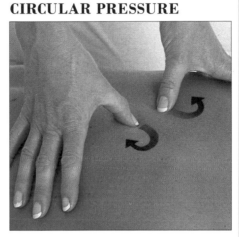

Press as for static pressure, then make small, penetrating, circular movements, circling the skin against the underlying muscle.

KNUCKLING

These small circling strokes give a rippling effect. Use them on the shoulders and chest, and on the palms of the hands and soles of the feet.

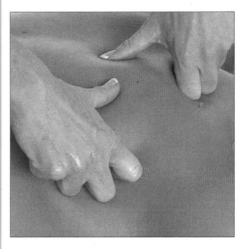

Curl your hands into loose fists and, with the middle section of your fingers against the skin, ripple your fingers round in a circular movement.

PERCUSSION

Brisk, bouncy percussion movements are useful on fleshy, muscular areas. Never use them on bony areas or over broken veins or bruises. They improve the circulation and are generally very stimulating, though if performed more slowly, they can be calming. Use them at the end of a massage to wake the person up; if you are trying to send someone to sleep, omit them altogether or do them earlier in the massage. Keep the movements light and springy rather than heavy and pounding. Practise on yourself, or do the movements over a towel at first, to avoid hurting your friend.

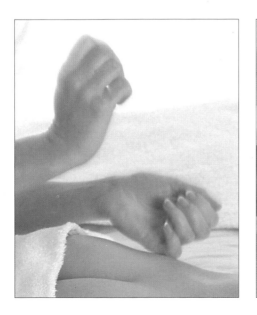

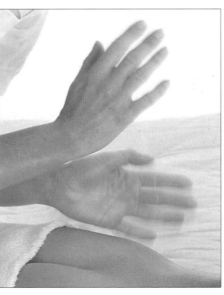

PUMMELLING ◄◄

Make your hands into loose fists and, with relaxed wrists, bounce the side of your fists alternately against the skin. Pull your hands away as soon as you touch the skin, so that the movement feels light and bouncy rather than heavy and thumping.

HACKING ◄

Strike the skin with the side of your hands, flicking them away just as you touch the skin. Use your hands alternately, and work very quickly. Your hands should be completely relaxed, so that you can hear your fingers knocking together.

AROMATHERAPY

The use of aromatic extracts from plants can add a whole new dimension to your massage. These concentrated essences, taken from flowers, herbs and trees, are known as essential oils. Aromatherapy is the practice of using these oils therapeutically to treat a wide range of problems from insomnia and stress to acne, ageing skin, depression and nervous tension.

THE POWER OF SCENT

People usually don't realize how strongly they are affected by scents. Yet the evocative power of a scent is dramatic – the smell of the sea or of your mother's perfume can bring memories rushing back. The reason for this is that smells are interpreted by the area of the brain that is concerned with our emotions. Scents have a powerful effect on our moods, so adding some essential oils to your massage oil can enhance the relaxing or invigorating effect of your massage.

Recent research testifies to the strength of this link. Dr Gary Schwartz, professor of psychology and psychiatry at Yale University, has found that certain odours can lower blood pressure. The scent of spiced apples was shown to be particularly effective: it lowered the blood pressure of healthy volunteers by an average of three to five points. Other scientific research has demonstrated that pleasant smells such as plum or peach can reduce pain, and that essential oils can change people's moods: jasmine, ylang ylang and peppermint can lift depression, geranium and bergamot dispel anxiety, and rose and carnation restore energy.

THERAPEUTIC USES

Essential oils are a complex mixture of chemicals with many different properties. As well as affecting mood, some are antibacterial, antiseptic or anti-inflammatory. The chart on page 20 lists some of the most common oils with the properties ascribed to them.

The diversity of claims made for essential oils, sometimes several claims for one oil, can cause confusion. A single oil may be described as both calming and stimulating. This sounds like a contradiction, causing sceptics to dismiss the whole subject. However, someone suffering from nervous tension might first be calmed by the treatment, and then, with this new freedom from tension, reclaim his natural energy and feel refreshed and energized.

HISTORY

"The way to health is to have an aromatic bath and scented massage every day," wrote Hippocrates in 400 BC. There are numerous references throughout history to the use of aromatic oils.

The term aromatherapy was coined by a French chemist, Gattefosse, in the 1920s. Several years earlier he had noticed the therapeutic effects of essential oils after burning his hand badly while working in his laboratory. Absent-mindedly, he put his burnt hand into the nearest liquid, a bowl of lavender oil. To his amazement, the pain diminished and the burn healed much faster than he expected, leaving no scar. Following this discovery, when working with wounded soldiers during the 1914-18 war, he found that essential oils accelerated the healing process. Since then, aromatherapy has steadily gained in popularity.

BUYING ESSENTIAL OILS

The price of essential oils varies greatly: for a small quantity of lavender oil, you would

ESSENTIAL OILS blended with your massage oil will impart a feeling of luxury to the massage. They perfume the oil and can help to relax or refresh.

pay only a tiny fraction of the cost of the same amount of rose oil. This reflects the fact that it takes about 200 kilos (over 30 stone) of rose petals to produce just a litre ($1\frac{3}{4}$ pints) of rose oil, whereas 200 kilos of lavender flowers yield about six litres (10 or 11 pints) of essential oil.

The quality of the oil also varies considerably, depending partly on the process used to extract the oil from the plant, and partly on whether the oil is adulterated with a similar smelling, but cheaper, oil. For aromatherapy you should use top quality oils.

BLENDING OILS

Essential oils are extremely concentrated and must always be diluted, otherwise they can sting and even cause allergies. To use them during a massage, you need to dilute them in a carrier oil. The most commonly used carrier oils are almond, soya, grapeseed, avocado, peach and wheatgerm oils. Wheatgerm oil is rich in vitamin E and acts as an antioxidant, but it is rather thick

and heavy, so add just a little to a lighter carrier oil to prevent your massage oil turning rancid.

To dilute an essential oil, mix one to three drops with a 5ml teaspoon of carrier oil. If you want to make up a larger quantity, add 15 to 30 drops to 50ml (2fl oz) of carrier oil. Use a more dilute mixture on sensitive skin and on the face. Don't mix much more than this at a time, as the blended oil can turn rancid in a few weeks. Despite their name, essential oils are usually not very oily; they are exceptionally volatile liquids which evaporate quickly, so always put the lids back on the bottles after use. Store them and your blended massage oil in a cool, dark place in air-tight bottles.

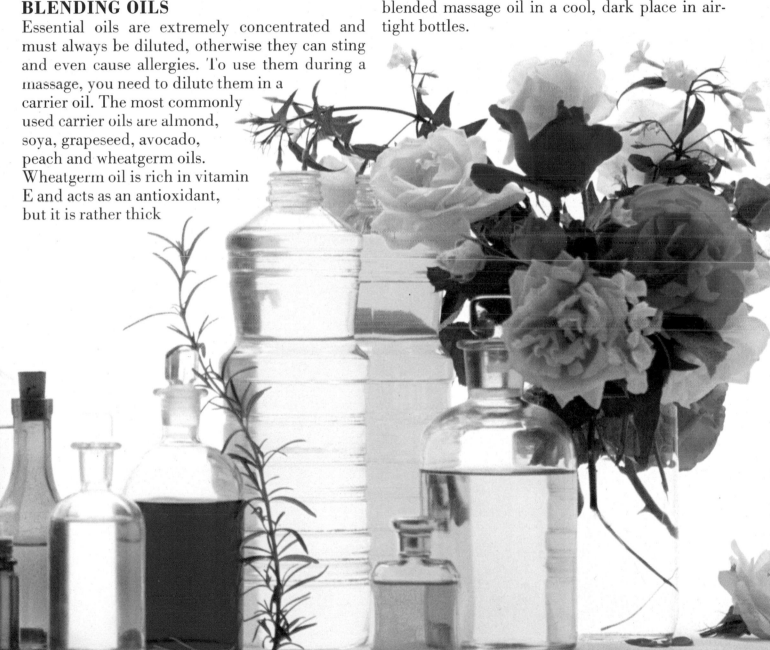

CHOOSING ESSENTIAL OILS

All essential oils add a feeling of luxury to a massage, so choose any that appeal to you. These are some of the most common essential oils and the properties ascribed to them. In perfumery, fragrances are categorized into different "notes" according to how quickly they evaporate. A top note evaporates very quickly and makes the initial impact, a middle note is mellow, and a base note is long lasting. If you blend essential oils, it is a good idea to choose an oil in each category so that the fragrance lasts throughout the massage.

OIL	FRAGRANCE	NOTE	PROPERTIES
BERGAMOT	Fresh and sharp	Middle	Antiseptic, astringent, antidepressant. Used for acne and greasy skin or hair. Sensitizes the skin to ultra-violet light, so do not use just before sunbathing.
CHAMOMILE	Fruity, apple-like	Middle	Calming, soothes the nerves. Suitable for sensitive skins. Used in hair products to lighten blond hair.
CLARY SAGE	Green	Top	Astringent, stimulating. Used as a fixative in perfumes; an ingredient of eau de Cologne.
EUCALYPTUS	Fresh and tangy	Top	Antiseptic and stimulating. Used for treating coughs and colds, and aching.
FRANKINCENSE	Woody	Base	Calming, aids relaxation, treats respiratory problems. Said to combat wrinkles.
GERANIUM	Sharp and flowery	Middle	Astringent, diuretic, antidepressant. Tones the skin, helps to blend a fragrance, and acts as an insect repellant.
JASMINE	Exotic and sweet	Base	Antidepressant, aphrodisiac, said to speed up labour. Good for treating postnatal depression.
LAVENDER	Fresh	Middle	Antiseptic, analgesic, calming. Treats headaches, insomnia, depression, aches, pains, wounds, insect bites.
MARJORAM	Green	Middle	Analgesic, sedative, warming, comforting. Treats aches and pains, period pains, insomnia and headaches. Increases local blood circulation, so useful after exercise.
NEROLI (orange blossom)	Sweet	Middle	Sedative, calming, aphrodisiac. Helps anxiety and insomnia. Especially suitable for dry skin.
PETITGRAIN (leaves of the bitter orange)	Sweet	Middle	Sedative, calming and refreshing. Treats anxiety and insomnia. Known as "poor man's neroli".
ROSE	Sweet and luxurious	Base	Antiseptic, sedative, antidepressant. Extremely expensive, but only a little is needed to add its distinctive fragrance.
ROSEMARY	Sharp and herby	Middle	Stimulating, helps memory and clear thinking. Treats rheumatic pain, and aches and pains after exercise. Used in shampoo and hair conditioner to enrich dark hair.
SANDALWOOD	Exotic and luxurious	Base	Antiseptic, sedative, calming, aphrodisiac. Suitable for dry, dehydrated skin and, because it is antiseptic, used on acne. Helps to blend a fragrance.
TEA TREE OIL	Sharp and spicy	Top	Antiseptic, germicidal, fungicidal, soothing and healing. Treats cuts, burns, infections, pimples and boils.
YLANG YLANG	Exotic and sweet	Base	Antidepressant, sedative, antiseptic, aphrodisiac. Allays anxiety, good for problem and oily skins.

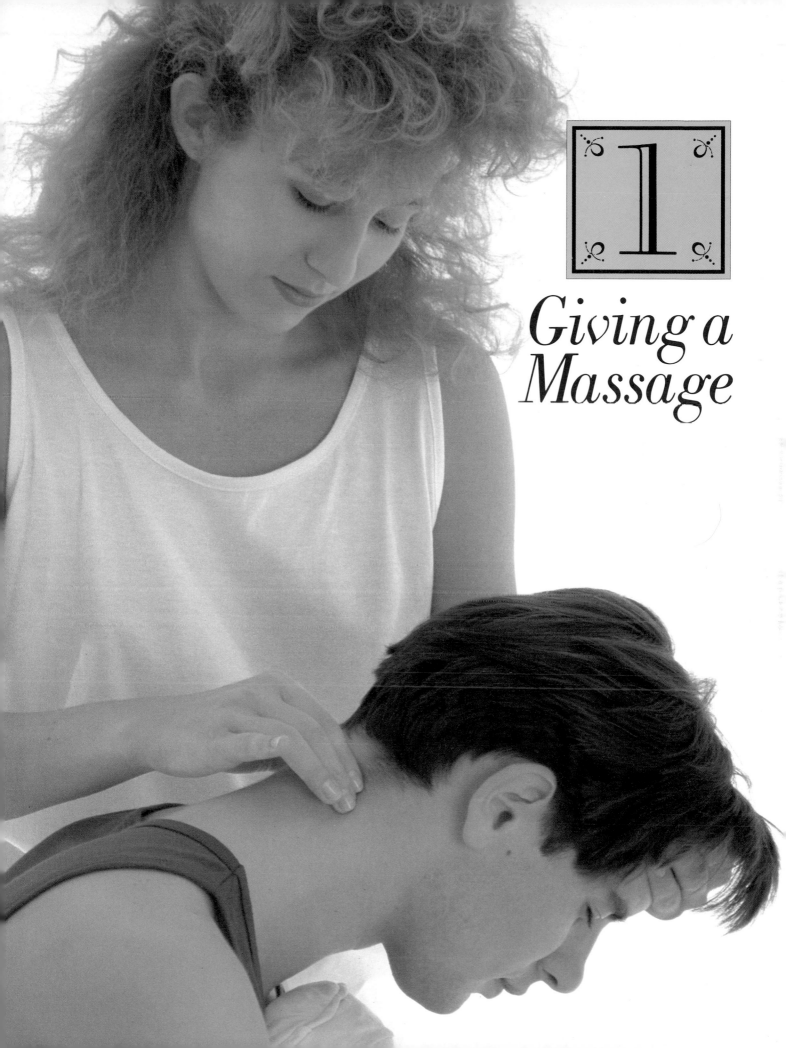

1

Giving a Massage

BACK MASSAGE

A good back massage can be one of the great delights of life. It can have a profoundly relaxing effect, lowering stress levels, easing pain and inducing a blissful state of repose.

Most of us get the occasional backache: we slouch over our desks, carry heavy loads, hunch up our shoulders and stand badly, all of which may result in tense, knotted muscles. Massage can help to relax these muscles and alleviate the aches and pains they so often cause.

The benefits of a back massage go beyond simply relaxing the back muscles. A good back massage enhances the well-being of the whole body. Nerves branch out from the spine to reach all parts of the body, and through its direct effect on them, massage can benefit the entire nervous system. You can calm the nerves with slow, rhythmic strokes, or invigorate them with fast, brisk movements. I usually finish with soothing strokes, to leave the person thoroughly relaxed.

INITIAL TOUCH

Cover your friend's back with a towel and place your hands on it, one on the nape of the neck and the other on the waist. Breathe deeply and evenly, and focus your attention on your hands.

This sets the tone for your massage and helps both of you to relax. Your friend will pick up your breathing rhythm and will start to relax automatically. As you breathe deeply and relax, you will begin to feel energy flowing through you, and it is this relaxed energy that you will use during the massage.

After about 30 seconds put the oil on your hands and pull back the towel. Kneel by the side of the waist, facing towards the head, and begin the massage by stroking to spread the oil.

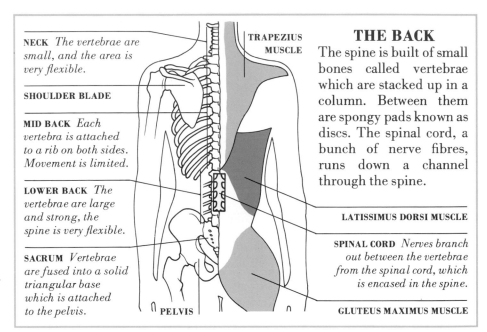

NECK *The vertebrae are small, and the area is very flexible.*

SHOULDER BLADE

MID BACK *Each vertebra is attached to a rib on both sides. Movement is limited.*

LOWER BACK *The vertebrae are large and strong, the spine is very flexible.*

SACRUM *Vertebrae are fused into a solid triangular base which is attached to the pelvis.*

PELVIS

TRAPEZIUS MUSCLE

THE BACK

The spine is built of small bones called vertebrae which are stacked up in a column. Between them are spongy pads known as discs. The spinal cord, a bunch of nerve fibres, runs down a channel through the spine.

LATISSIMUS DORSI MUSCLE

SPINAL CORD *Nerves branch out between the vertebrae from the spinal cord, which is encased in the spine.*

GLUTEUS MAXIMUS MUSCLE

STROKING

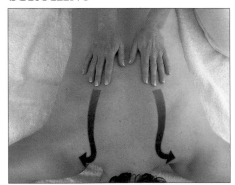

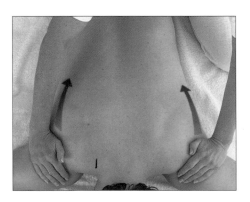

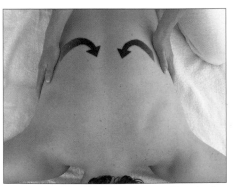

1 Start with your hands on the lower back, your thumbs on either side of the spine and your fingers pointing towards the head. With relaxed hands, stroke firmly up the back. Lean onto your hands, using your body weight to apply pressure.

2 Pull back down on the muscles at the base of the neck, then stroke out across the shoulders and the top of the arms, moulding your hands to the curve of the shoulders. Sweep your hands round the top of the arms and then down the sides.

3 Glide your hands lightly down the sides of the body, keeping them relaxed and taking care not to drag the skin. When you reach the waist, pull upwards and inwards. This gives the lovely feeling of having a tiny waist. Repeat up to ten times.

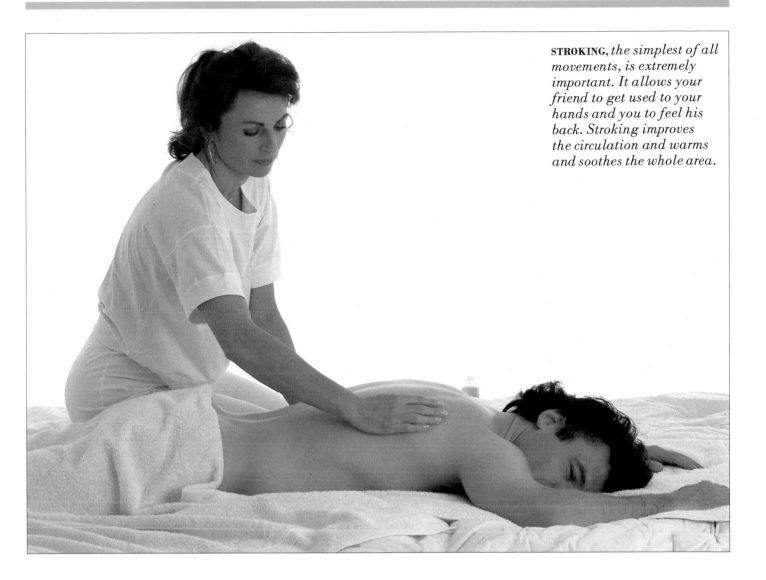

STROKING, *the simplest of all movements, is extremely important. It allows your friend to get used to your hands and you to feel his back. Stroking improves the circulation and warms and soothes the whole area.*

FAN STROKING

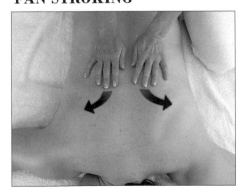

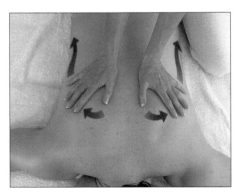

ALTERNATE STROKING

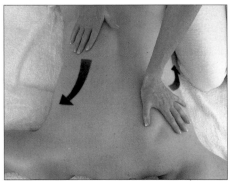

1 This movement is very similar to the first stroking, but the slight variation makes the massage more interesting. Start with your hands on the lower back, as before, and stroke firmly up the back, pressing on the muscles on either side of the spine.

2 Fan your hands out over the lower ribs, moulding them to the contours of the body, and glide them lightly down the sides. Repeat the stroke, fanning your hands out a little higher on the back each time, until you reach the shoulders.

Continue stroking the back, but use your hands alternately. One hand strokes firmly upwards as the other glides down the side. Practise this until it is smooth and rhythmic. When done properly, it is a wonderful continuous flowing stroke.

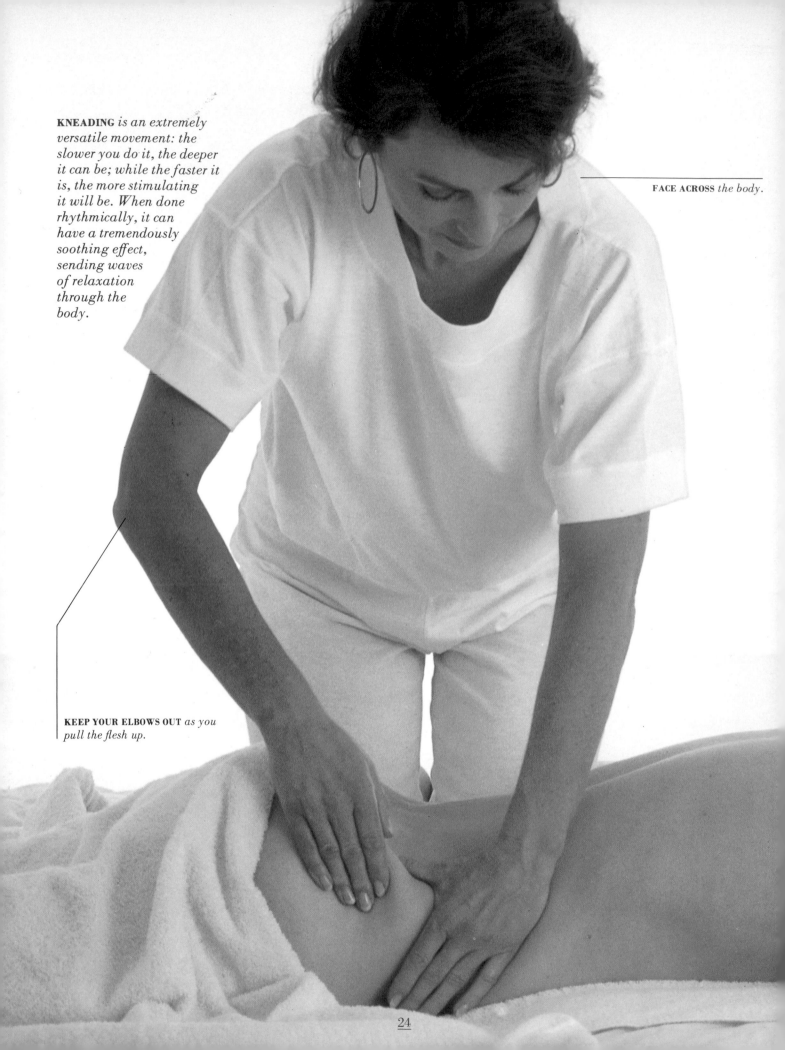

KNEADING *is an extremely versatile movement: the slower you do it, the deeper it can be; while the faster it is, the more stimulating it will be. When done rhythmically, it can have a tremendously soothing effect, sending waves of relaxation through the body.*

FACE ACROSS *the body.*

KEEP YOUR ELBOWS OUT *as you pull the flesh up.*

KNEADING

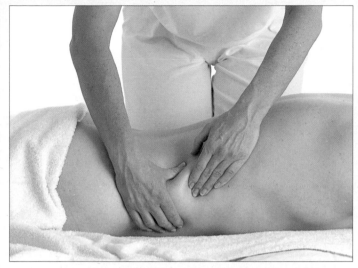

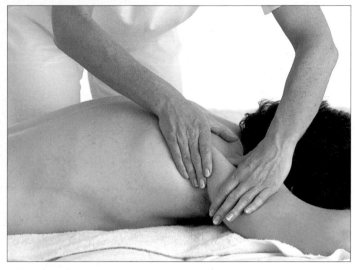

1 Turn to face across the body, and with your hands facing each other and your elbows out, grasp and squeeze handfuls of flesh with alternate hands. It is just like rhythmically kneading dough, but the movement must be smooth and flowing. Grasp the flesh with one hand, squeeze it, but do not pinch, and push it towards the other hand. Release the first hand, then pick up and squeeze the flesh with the second hand. Start at the hips and work up the sides of the body.

2 Continue kneading at the base of the neck, over the shoulders and out across the upper arms. The muscle at the top of the arms is often very tense, and since it is continuous with the large muscle across the upper back, you need to include the area in the massage in order to relax the back thoroughly. Then work on the side nearest you – either lean down so that you can push up with your thumbs, or move to the other side of the body and reach across again. Work your way round the back twice.

SIDE STROKING

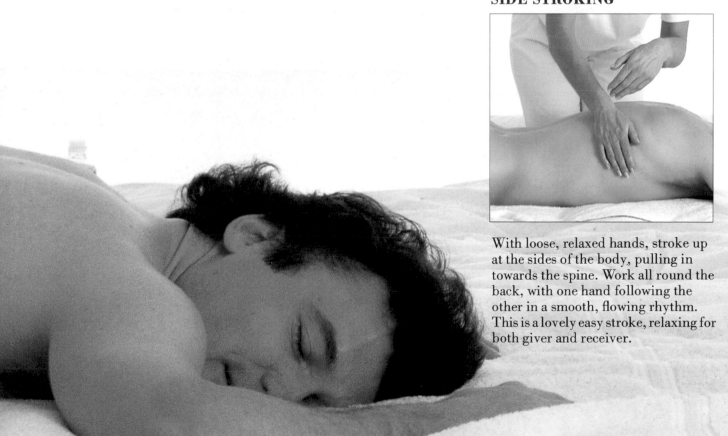

With loose, relaxed hands, stroke up at the sides of the body, pulling in towards the spine. Work all round the back, with one hand following the other in a smooth, flowing rhythm. This is a lovely easy stroke, relaxing for both giver and receiver.

CIRCLE STROKING

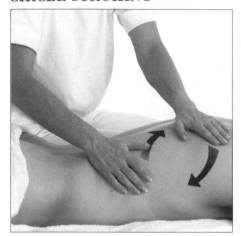

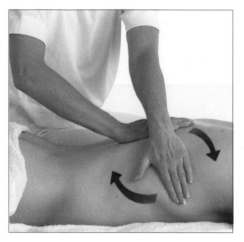

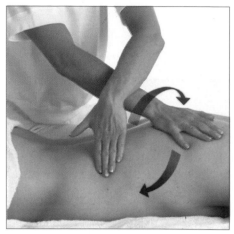

1 Place both hands on the right-hand side of the back, one a little higher than the other. Slide the top hand down the side in a large curve, and the lower hand up to the spine.

2 Continue stroking round in these wide curves. Imagine a circle on the back, and stroke round the circle in a clockwise direction, one hand following the other.

3 Lift your left hand over your right arm while your right hand continues stroking. Your right hand does a complete circle and your left hand does only a half circle.

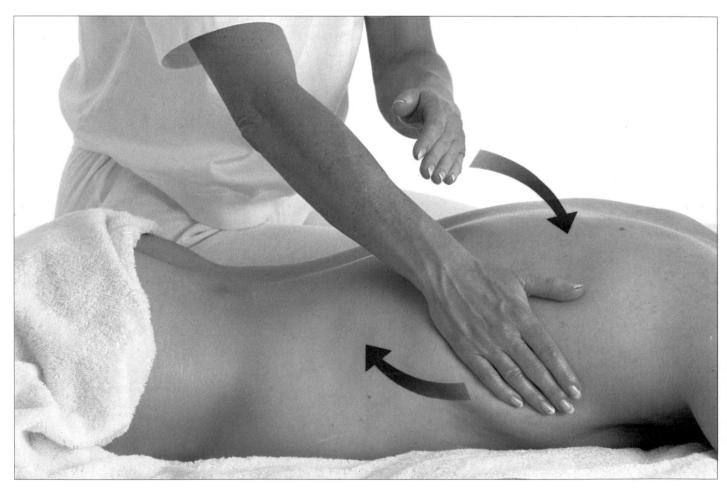

4 Complete the circle with your right hand and place your left hand down gently. Work up the back on this side, then slide your hands down and work on the lefthand side: stroke anti-clockwise round the circle, with your left hand doing the complete circle. This continuous, flowing stroke sends people off into a dream-like state.

PRESSURES

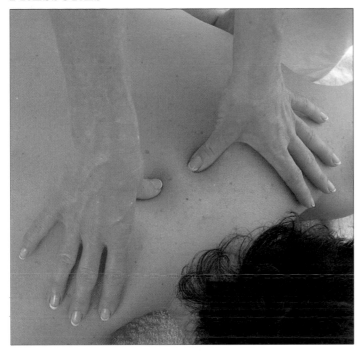

You can relax the small muscles on either side of the spine with a series of firm pressures. Start at the lower back, with your thumbs on either side of the spine. Lean your weight onto the pad of your thumbs, keeping your elbows straight, to apply a relaxed pressure, not a sharp poke. Press firmly, then release and repeat a little further up. Do extra work on the shoulders and the base of the neck, then glide back to the base of the spine and start again. Vary the movement by making small, penetrating circles over these muscles.

FINGER DRUMMING

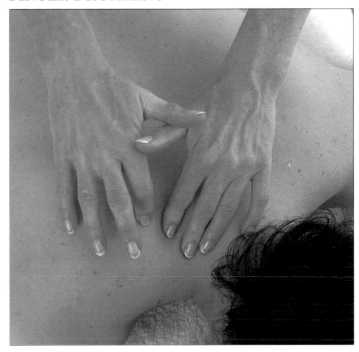

This is a strange movement, and it can be rather tiring since it is the only time when you cannot use your body weight – you just use the strength of your hands. It is particularly useful on the shoulder muscles. Drum your fingers down individually, pressing heavily on the muscle. Keep your hands close together and if, like me, one hand is stronger than the other, cross your thumbs to equalize the pressure. This heavy drumming movement brings blood to the area and eases away pain.

CIRCLE THUMB STROKING

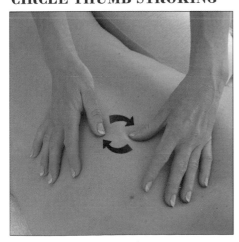

1 This is similar to the circle stroking opposite, but the movement is much smaller. Start with both thumbs on one side of the spine and stroke round in a circle.

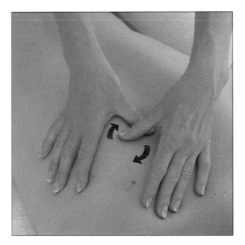

2 One thumb follows the other as you stroke up and out, pushing the muscle away from the spine. The movement is quite precise, working about an inch from the spine.

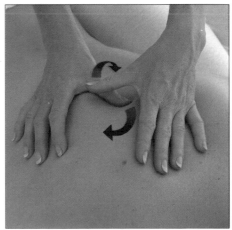

3 Lift one thumb over the other hand and continue circling. As for circle stroking, one thumb makes a complete circle, and the other just does a half circle.

THE NECK AND SHOULDERS

Always give extra attention to the neck, because the area is so often stiff and tense. This is hardly surprising, since the neck muscles have to work continuously to support the head – which weighs between five and seven kilos (about a stone). Many people habitually hunch their shoulders, making the muscles at the sides of the neck very tense.

If your friend is not comfortable with his head turned to one side, he can lie face down with a small cushion or rolled towel under his forehead.

STROKING

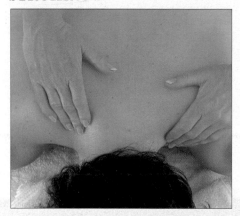

1 Stroke from the top of the shoulders up the sides of the neck, moulding your hands to the shape of the body.

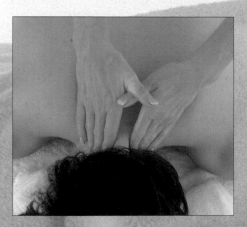

2 Reach right to the top of the neck, then glide your hands down, keeping the pressure smooth and even. Repeat about four times.

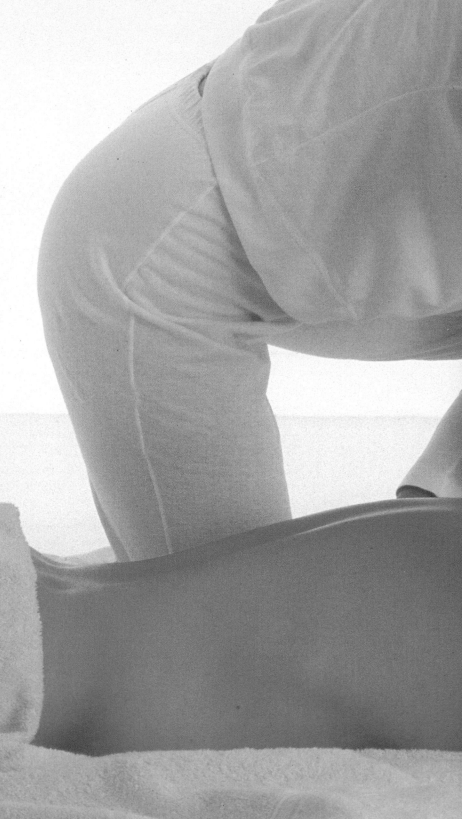

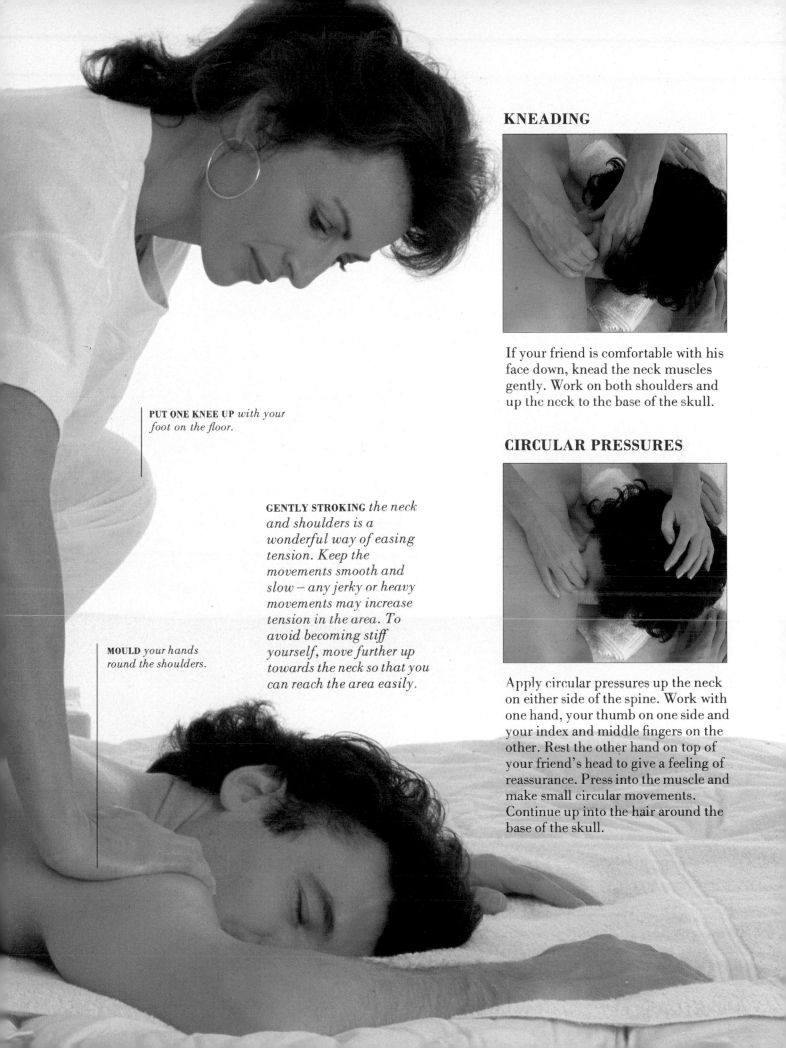

PUT ONE KNEE UP *with your foot on the floor.*

KNEADING

If your friend is comfortable with his face down, knead the neck muscles gently. Work on both shoulders and up the neck to the base of the skull.

CIRCULAR PRESSURES

Apply circular pressures up the neck on either side of the spine. Work with one hand, your thumb on one side and your index and middle fingers on the other. Rest the other hand on top of your friend's head to give a feeling of reassurance. Press into the muscle and make small circular movements. Continue up into the hair around the base of the skull.

GENTLY STROKING the neck and shoulders is a wonderful way of easing tension. Keep the movements smooth and slow – any jerky or heavy movements may increase tension in the area. To avoid becoming stiff yourself, move further up towards the neck so that you can reach the area easily.

MOULD *your hands round the shoulders.*

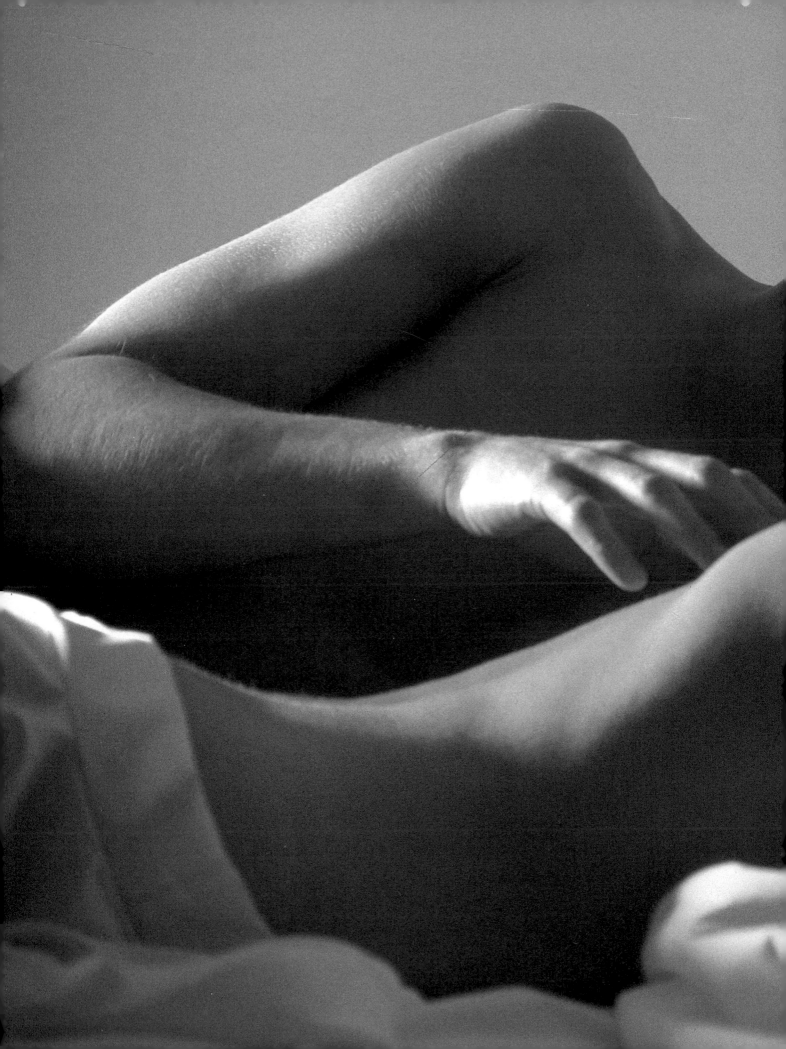

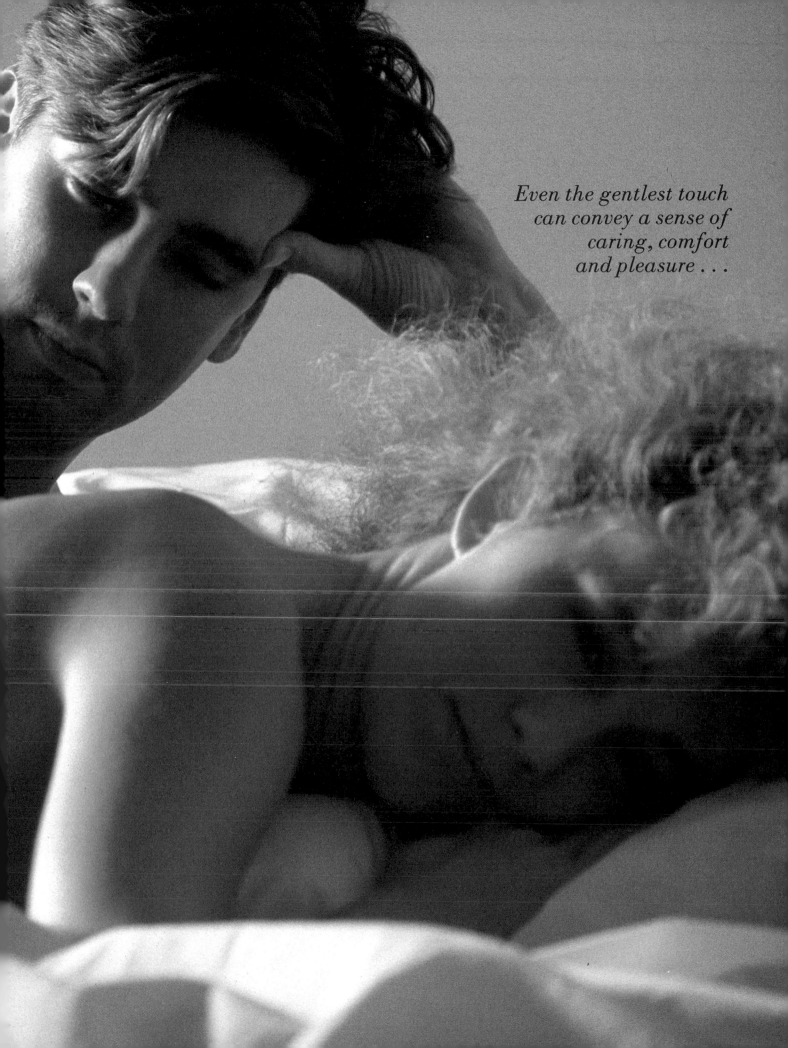

Even the gentlest touch can convey a sense of caring, comfort and pleasure . . .

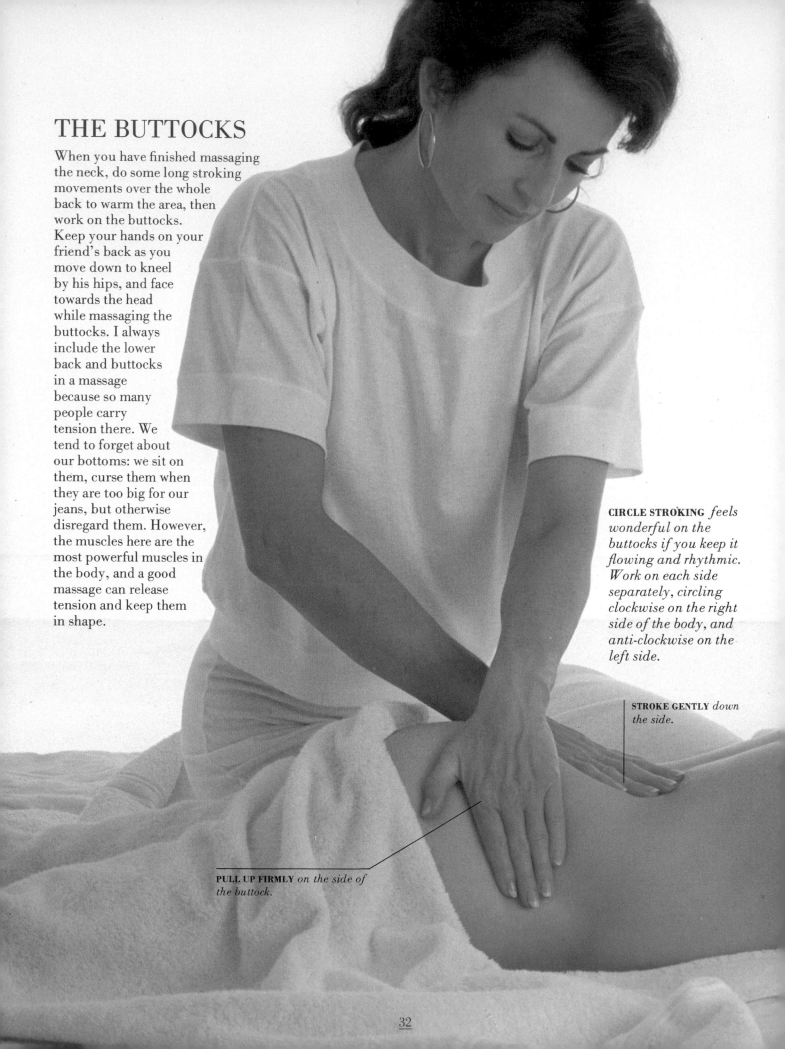

THE BUTTOCKS

When you have finished massaging the neck, do some long stroking movements over the whole back to warm the area, then work on the buttocks. Keep your hands on your friend's back as you move down to kneel by his hips, and face towards the head while massaging the buttocks. I always include the lower back and buttocks in a massage because so many people carry tension there. We tend to forget about our bottoms: we sit on them, curse them when they are too big for our jeans, but otherwise disregard them. However, the muscles here are the most powerful muscles in the body, and a good massage can release tension and keep them in shape.

CIRCLE STROKING *feels wonderful on the buttocks if you keep it flowing and rhythmic. Work on each side separately, circling clockwise on the right side of the body, and anti-clockwise on the left side.*

STROKE GENTLY *down the side.*

PULL UP FIRMLY *on the side of the buttock.*

FAN STROKING

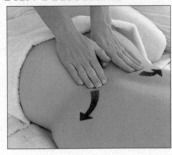

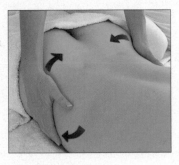

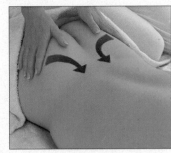

1 Place your hands at the top of the buttocks, and stroke smoothly up and out.

2 Keep your hands relaxed and mould them round the sides of the waist.

3 Pull firmly up at the sides, then swing your hands round and repeat.

KNEADING

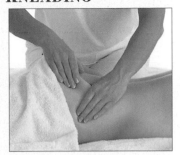

This fleshy area can take some deep kneading. Put a twist into the movement.

CIRCLE STROKING

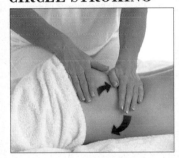

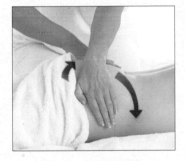

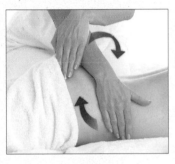

1 With both hands on one side, stroke round in a circle, one hand following the other, as on page 26.

2 Stroke gently as you glide down the sides, and pull firmly up at the buttocks.

3 Lift one hand over the other arm to complete the circle, and continue. Repeat on the other side.

PRESSURES

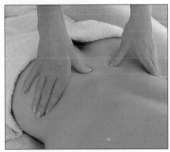

Apply circular pressures with your thumbs around the bony triangle at the base of the spine.

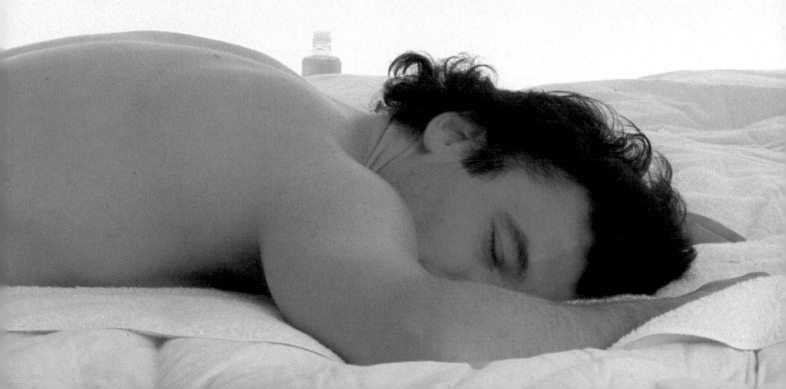

THE BACK

Now turn to face across the back and return to work on the main part of it to finish off the massage.

CRADLING

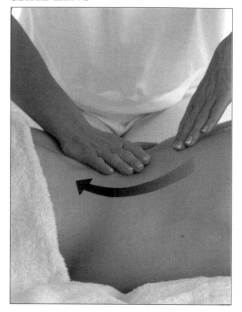

1 This is a warming, comforting movement. With relaxed hands facing each other, do some open-handed kneading on the lower back.

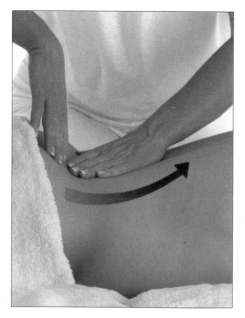

2 Do not grasp and squeeze the flesh, simply sway your hands back and forth in a deep, penetrating stroke.

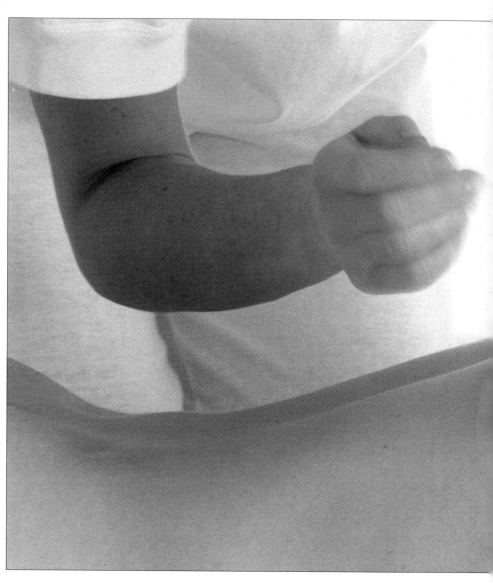

CRISS-CROSSING

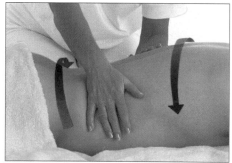

1 Put one hand on each side of the waist, with the fingers of both hands facing away from you. Pull your hands firmly up the sides of the body, gently pulling the waist in, and glide them across the back.

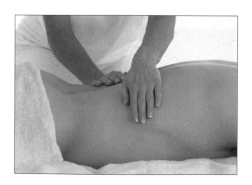

2 Slide your hands past each other and down the other side. Make a definite contrast between firmly pulling up the sides, and lightly gliding across the back. Work up and down the back a couple of times.

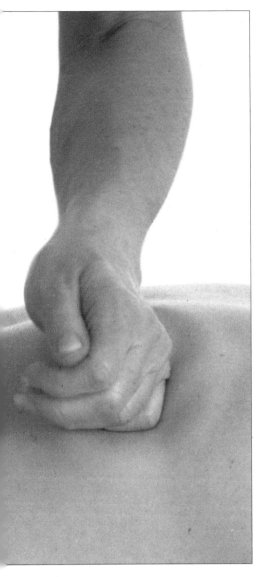

CAT STROKING

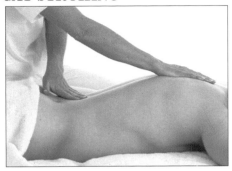

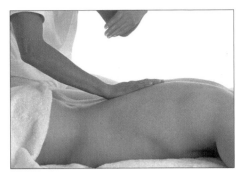

1 This smooth, continuous stroke calms the nerves and has a hypnotic, soporific effect. Start at the neck and stroke gently down the spine with one hand, and as it reaches the bottom, follow it with the other hand.

2 Lift your hand off at the small of the back and return it to the neck. The return movement is as important as the stroke itself, so move rhythmically. Gradually stroke more and more slowly and lightly.

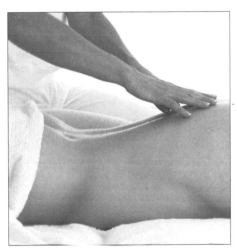

FEATHER TOUCH

When the cat stroke cannot become any lighter, move on to the feather touch. Stroke very, very lightly down either side of the spine with both hands together, using just your fingertips. At the small of the back lift your hands off and return them to the neck. Shake your hands gently between each stroke to keep them feeling light and to get rid of the feeling of electricity that tends to gather. The movement should be so smooth and rhythmic that it feels as though it has no beginning or end. Continue for as long as you like.

PUMMELLING▲

Make loose fists with your hands and pummel all over the back. Your wrists should be very flexible and loose so that the movement is light, springy and stimulating, not heavy and painful. Start on the buttocks and move up the back, avoiding the kidney area. Work more gently over bony areas, and never strike the spine itself. Vary the speed for different effects: slow for relaxation and vigorous for a stimulating effect. As this is the easiest, as well as the nicest, percussion movement, it is the best one for beginners. While you are learning, put a towel over your friend's back and pummel through that to avoid stinging.

THE FINAL TOUCH

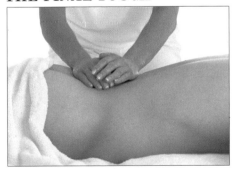

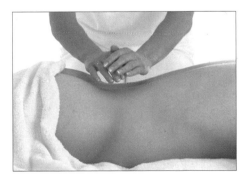

1 Finish the massage by placing relaxed, slightly cupped hands over the small of the back. Hold them there and feel heat gathering underneath. Ease the heat into the body by gently flattening your hands.

2 Lift your hands away very, very slowly. The movement should be so gentle that your friend does not know when your hands leave. This gives such a feeling of lightness that one friend calls it her "magic carpet".

EXTRA MOVEMENTS

You can include any of these movements in the back massage. Experiment to see which of them your friend enjoys.

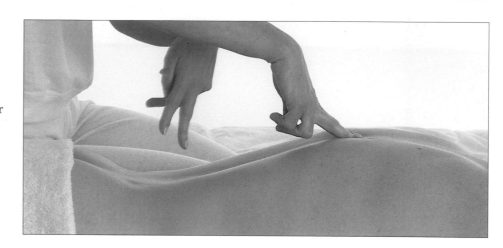

RAKING DOWN THE SPINE

Start at the neck with your index and middle fingers on either side of the spine. Make small, firm strokes down the back, one hand after the other.

CATERPILLAR WALKING

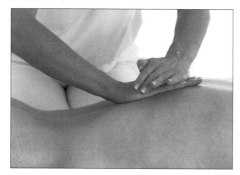 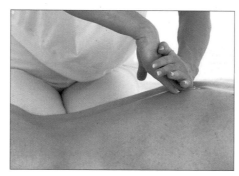 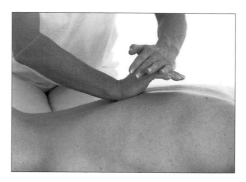

1 Place your right hand at the base of the spine, the middle of your palm resting on the bone, your ring and middle fingers straddling the spine. Put your left hand across the fingers.

2 Lift up the heel of your right hand and press your fingers down, adding depth with your left hand. Place the heel of the hand down again as close to your fingers as possible.

3 Lift up your fingers and move them up the back. Climb up the back with this bouncy, rocking movement. Though you are working over the spine, never press hard on the vertebrae.

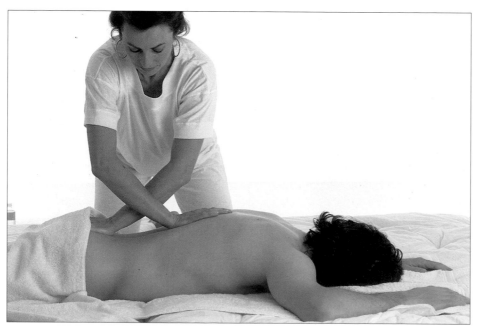

STRETCHING

A good way to begin or end a back massage is to give the back a gentle stretch. Cross your arms and place one hand on the sacrum and the other half way up the spine, with your hands facing away from each other. Lean forwards, keeping your arms rigid, and do not let your hands slip up or down the back. As you lean, the pressure of your arms being pushed apart stretches the lower back gently.

You can give a diagonal stretch to the back by placing one hand on your friend's shoulder and the other on the opposite hip, with your hands facing away from each other. Again, lean forwards, keeping your arms straight, to stretch the back. Repeat on the other shoulder and hip.

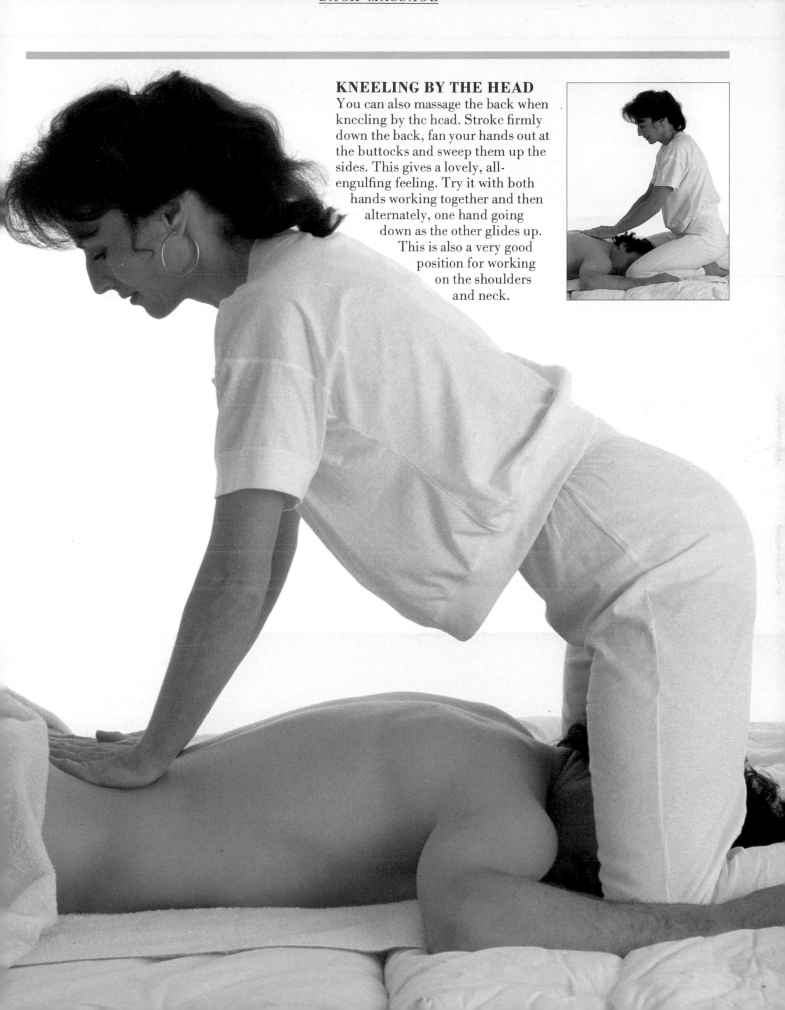

KNEELING BY THE HEAD
You can also massage the back when kneeling by the head. Stroke firmly down the back; fan your hands out at the buttocks and sweep them up the sides. This gives a lovely, all-engulfing feeling. Try it with both hands working together and then alternately, one hand going down as the other glides up. This is also a very good position for working on the shoulders and neck.

FOOT MASSAGE

Few things are more relaxing than a good foot massage. Tired feet suddenly feel light again and the whole body is refreshed. The foot, particularly the sole, contains thousands of nerve endings, and by massaging these you can stimulate the whole body. Regular foot massage helps to keep the feet flexible and healthy.

Kneel at the feet and work first on one foot, then on the other. You need very little oil: if you have too much, your fingers slide about, which can be rather ticklish. If your friend has ticklish feet, massage very firmly or work on the legs first. Ticklishness seems to be linked to tension, so if you return to ticklish feet after the leg massage, your friend may be sufficiently relaxed to enjoy the foot massage.

ANATOMY OF THE FEET

Leonardo da Vinci referred to the foot as "the greatest engineering device in the world". The feet contain almost a quarter of all the bones in the body: each has 28 separate bones and an intricate web of muscles. These bones are arranged in arches which help the foot to support the weight of the body and provide leverage when walking. There are three arches: the main, high arch runs along the inside edge of the foot, lower ones run along the outside edge and across the base of the toes. The sole has a thick layer of tough tissue covering many small ligaments and muscles. If the skin is very tough, your massage has to be extra firm to get through it.

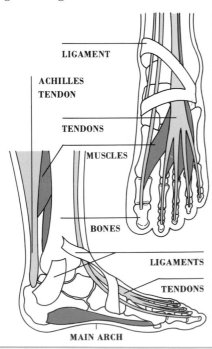

LIGAMENT

ACHILLES TENDON

TENDONS

MUSCLES

BONES

LIGAMENTS

TENDONS

MAIN ARCH

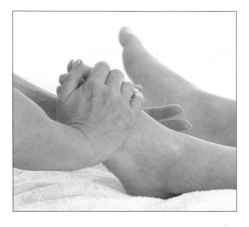

STROKING

1 ◀Start the massage by stroking the foot to get it used to your touch. Sandwich it between your hands and stroke firmly with both hands from the toes towards the body.

2 ▼When you reach the ankles, swing your hands round and return them to the toes with a light stroke. This is a warming movement, and is ideal for anyone who suffers from cold feet. Repeat at least four times.

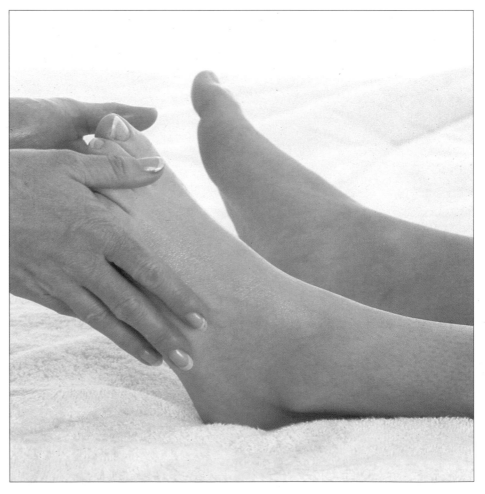

THUMB STROKING

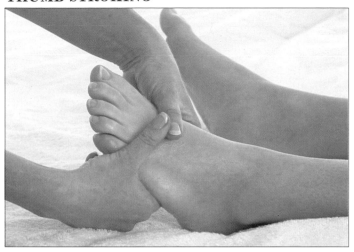

1 Support the foot with your fingers underneath it, and place your thumbs on top at the base of the toes. Stroke up the foot with your thumbs, fanning out to the sides and gliding back to the toes.

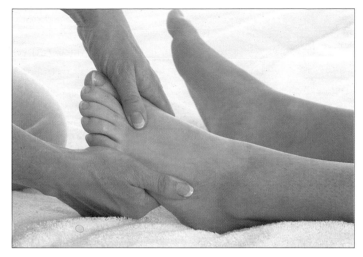

2 Now stroke with your thumbs working alternately. Stroke up with one thumb as the other glides back down the side. The movement can be a little longer than before, reaching up to the ankle.

TOE MASSAGE

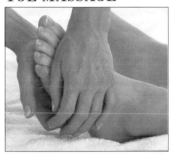

1 Loosen and warm the whole area by wiggling the toes. Sandwich the foot just above the toes and rotate your hands.

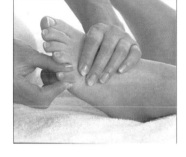

2 Massage each toe individually. Squeeze and roll it all over, rotate it in both directions, then pull it gently towards you.

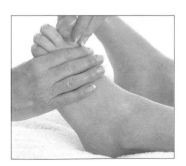

3 Change hands when you reach the big toe, and massage it very thoroughly. Then squeeze all round the base of the toe.

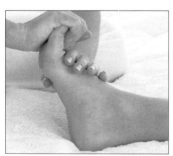

4 Clasp all the toes with one hand and then bend them gently backwards and forwards to encourage flexibility.

STROKING BETWEEN THE TENDONS

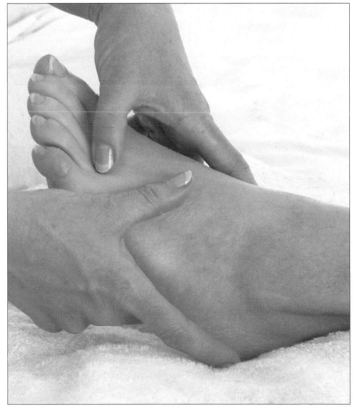

Support the foot with both hands, with your fingers underneath and your thumbs on top. Stroke in each furrow between the tendons, one thumb following the other. Run your thumbs up the foot towards the ankle, doing about four strokes in each furrow.

PRESSURES

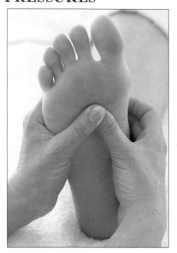

Support the foot with your fingers on top and your thumbs underneath. Press firmly on the sole with one thumb on top of the other for three to seven seconds, then move on about half an inch and repeat. Work all over the ball of the foot and in a line down the centre to the heel. Then do more pressures in lines on either side of this central line.

STROKE THE ARCH

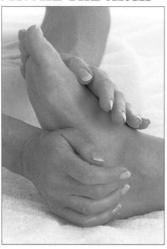

After that stimulating work, soothe the foot by stroking. Rest one hand on top of the foot and stroke firmly into the main arch, using the heel of your other hand. Curve your hand back to fit the shape of the foot, and stroke from the ball of the foot to the heel. Return with a light stroke to start again. Repeat at least four times.

KNUCKLING

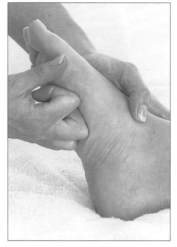

Keep one hand on top of the foot and curl the fingers of the other hand so that you can massage the foot with the middle section of your fingers. Move your fingers round to make rippling, rotary movements. Work firmly all over the sole. This feels wonderful, and is also very good for your hands, since it helps to keep them supple and flexible.

ROTARY PRESSURES

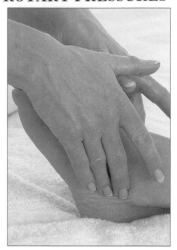

Stroke the whole foot as you did at the start, then apply circular pressures all round the ankle with one hand on each side. Press firmly on the upwards sweep of the circle, as you move towards the leg, and keep the pressure light on the return. Use your middle fingers on the sides and back of the ankle, then your thumbs on the front.

HACKING

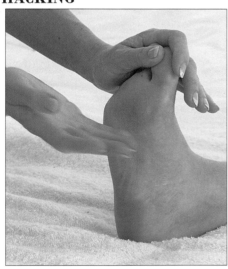

1 Hold the foot firmly with one hand, and hack the sole with the side of the other hand. The movement should be quick and light, so your hand must be very loose and flexible.

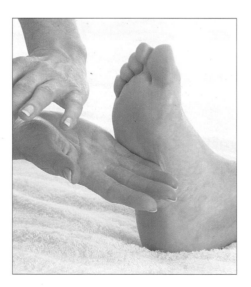

2 Now use both hands to hack the sole of the foot. This is an even faster movement. It is tremendously invigorating and feels wonderful. Use it when you want to wake someone up.

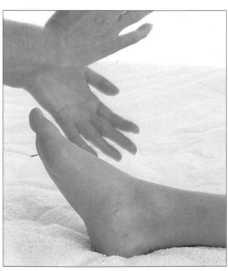

3 If you have a very light touch, you can also hack the top of the foot. Work gently, using both hands and make sure that your hands flick away as soon as they touch the foot.

STROKING

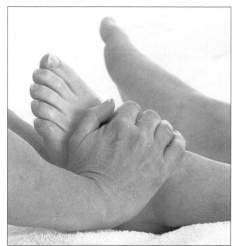

You are coming to the end of the foot massage, so stroke the whole foot to calm it down after the previous vigorous movement. Stroke with both hands up towards the ankle as you did at the beginning, then glide lightly back down. Finish by holding the foot for a few seconds, then gently slide your hands off the end of the toes.

THE FINAL TOUCH

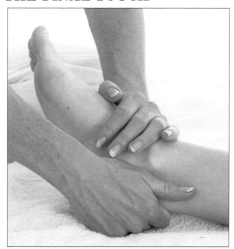

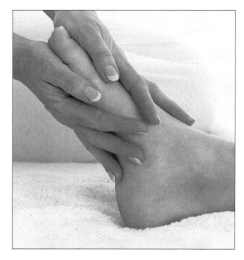

1 When you finish the massage, lift your hands away from the feet very slowly and gently. This sequence leaves the foot feeling soothed and cared for. Clasp the back of the ankle with your right hand and rest the other hand on top of the foot. Gently pull the leg towards you. Don't lift the leg up, just stretch it gently.

2 Release the stretch and slide your right hand under the foot. Hold the foot for about five seconds.

3 ▼Glide your hands towards the toes, moulding them to the shape of the foot. Slide them very, very slowly off the end of the toes. Repeat two or three times.

PASSIVE MOVEMENTS

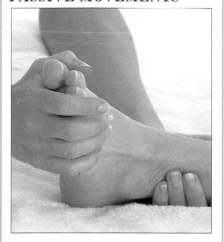

Towards the end of the massage, loosen the whole foot and ankle with gentle passive movements. Support the ankle with one hand, and with the other slowly flex the foot up and down. Hold at its furthest point for a count of four. Now turn the foot to each side, and finally rotate it about four times in each direction.

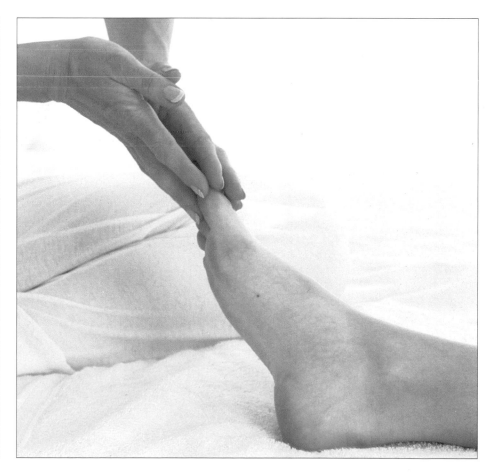

LEG MASSAGE

Everyone can benefit from a leg massage, whether they lead a sedentary or an active life. By stimulating the circulation, massage brings blood and nutrients to the legs and helps to prevent varicose veins. More active people can use leg massage as a warm-up before exercise and to get rid of tightness or cramp in the muscles afterwards. Deep, firm massage on the large muscles will help to dispel fatigue.

When massaging the legs, press very lightly over the bony areas, especially the shins and the knees. If your friend shows any sign of varicose veins, massage very gently, avoiding all heavy movements such as kneading and pummelling, and never press on the affected vein itself (see also page 134).

There are lymph nodes (see page 141) at the back of the knees and in the groin. Gentle stroking up the legs towards these nodes can help to reduce puffiness or swelling in the lower legs.

Backache can be caused or aggravated by problems in the legs. If your friend suffers from backache, you may be able to ease the pain by massaging the legs or feet.

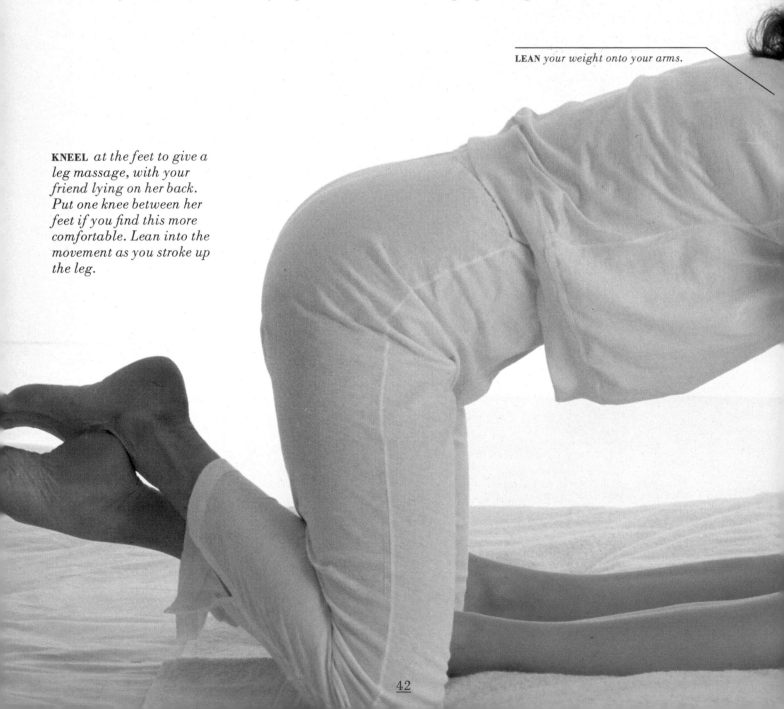

LEAN *your weight onto your arms.*

KNEEL *at the feet to give a leg massage, with your friend lying on her back. Put one knee between her feet if you find this more comfortable. Lean into the movement as you stroke up the leg.*

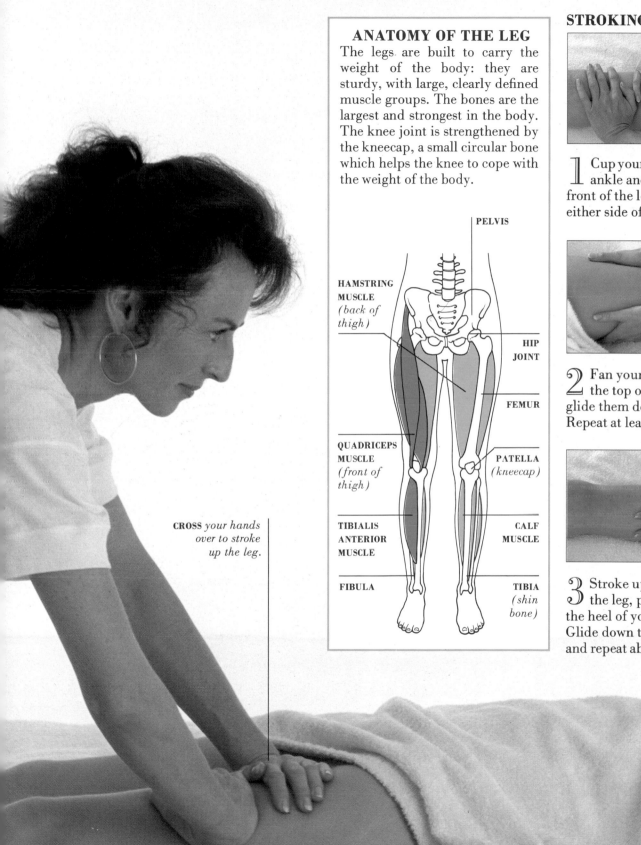

CROSS *your hands over to stroke up the leg.*

ANATOMY OF THE LEG

The legs are built to carry the weight of the body: they are sturdy, with large, clearly defined muscle groups. The bones are the largest and strongest in the body. The knee joint is strengthened by the kneecap, a small circular bone which helps the knee to cope with the weight of the body.

PELVIS

HAMSTRING MUSCLE *(back of thigh)*

HIP JOINT

FEMUR

QUADRICEPS MUSCLE *(front of thigh)*

PATELLA *(kneecap)*

TIBIALIS ANTERIOR MUSCLE

CALF MUSCLE

FIBULA

TIBIA *(shin bone)*

STROKING

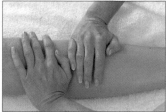

1 Cup your hands over the ankle and stroke up the front of the leg, pressing on either side of the bone.

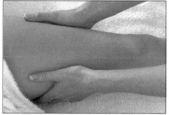

2 Fan your hands out at the top of the thigh and glide them down the sides. Repeat at least four times.

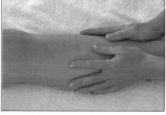

3 Stroke up the sides of the leg, pressing with the heel of your hands. Glide down to the ankle and repeat about four times.

KNEADING THE CALF

Support the ankle with one hand, and knead the calf muscle with the other. Squeeze and release the muscle, pressing the flesh between your palm and fingers. Knead the muscle away from the bone, pushing it upwards and outwards, and gradually working up the leg. When you reach the knee, release the pressure and glide back down to the ankle. Repeat a couple of times on one side, then change hands and knead the other side of the calf.

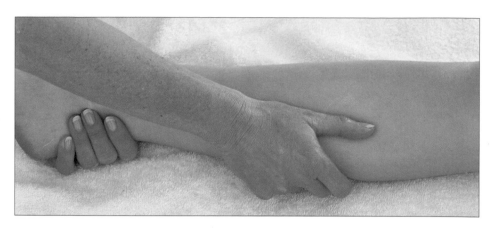

ALTERNATE STROKING UP THE CALF

Support your friend's ankle and bend her knee to rest her foot on the towel. Working with alternate hands, stroke firmly up the calf, then glide your hand back as the other strokes up. Stroke firmly, pulling the muscle up and out to the side. The movement should feel smooth and continuous. You will find it easier to get more rhythm into the stroke if you keep your elbows out to the sides. Anchor the foot to prevent the leg flopping around: if you are working on the floor, hold the foot between your knees; if you are working on a table, sit on the foot.

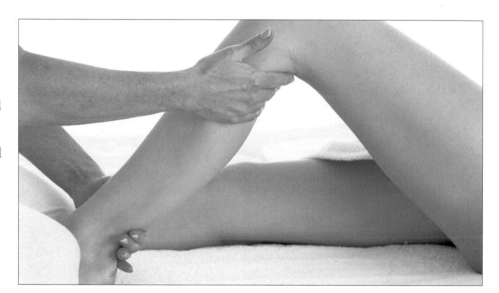

CRISS-CROSSING THE CALF

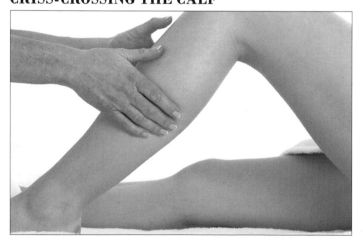

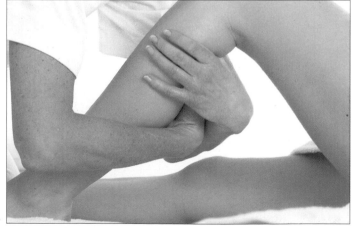

1 Anyone who does a lot of sport or who stands for hours at a time is likely to appreciate this movement, as it releases tension in the calf muscle. Never do it on legs with varicose veins. Place your hands round the leg, with your thumbs at the front and your fingers on the sides.

2 Slide your fingers round the calf, keeping the whole of your hands in contact with the skin. Release the pressure as your hands glide past each other. Work from the ankle to the knees and then back again, taking care not to pinch the flesh.

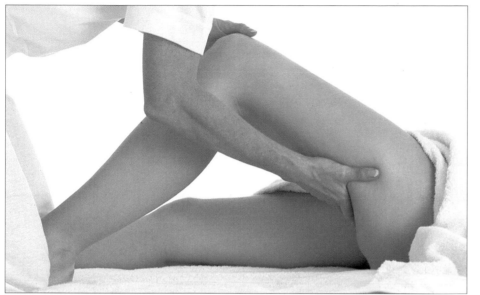

CRISS-CROSSING THE THIGH

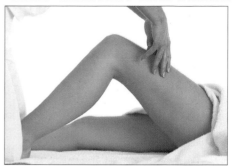

1 Now do some criss-crossing behind the thigh. Place your hands on top of the thigh, with your fingers curling round the sides.

2 ▼Squeeze the muscle by gliding your hands round under the thigh. Work up and down the thigh, then lower the leg onto the towel, supporting it at the knee and ankle. Stroke the whole leg a couple of times.

STROKING THE THIGH

With the leg still bent, lean forwards and stroke up the back of the thigh. As usual, stroke firmly towards the body and glide back down to the knee. Stroke with your hands working together, then alternately, one hand stroking up as the other glides back.

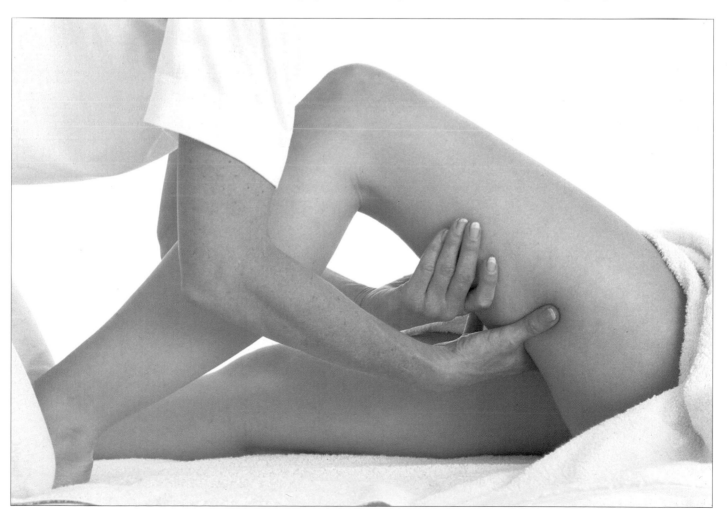

THUMB CIRCLING

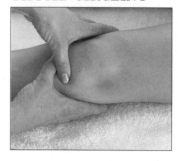 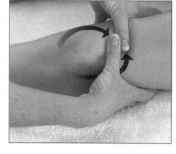 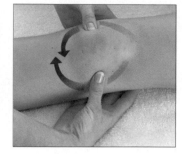

1 Now work on the knee. Support it with your fingers, and start with your thumbs crossed just underneath the knee.

2 Stroke gently up the sides of the knee to the top, one thumb on each side. Let your thumbs pass each other at the top.

3 Glide each thumb down the opposite side. Both thumbs do a complete circle, passing the other at the top and bottom.

ROTARY PRESSURES

STROKING

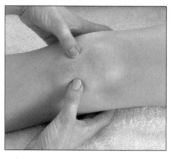 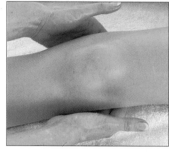

With your fingers behind the knee, make gentle rotary pressures with your thumbs all round the knee. Again, start below the knee and work all round it.

Stroke gently behind the knee with your fingers. Stroke up towards the body, then make gentle rotary movements behind the knee.

THE THIGHS *are an ideal place for fast, stimulating movements such as pummelling. Nearly all women love to have their thighs massaged, and kneading and pummelling can help to improve the shape of the thighs by smoothing down unsightly lumps and bumps.*

KNEEL *alongside the legs to massage the thighs.*

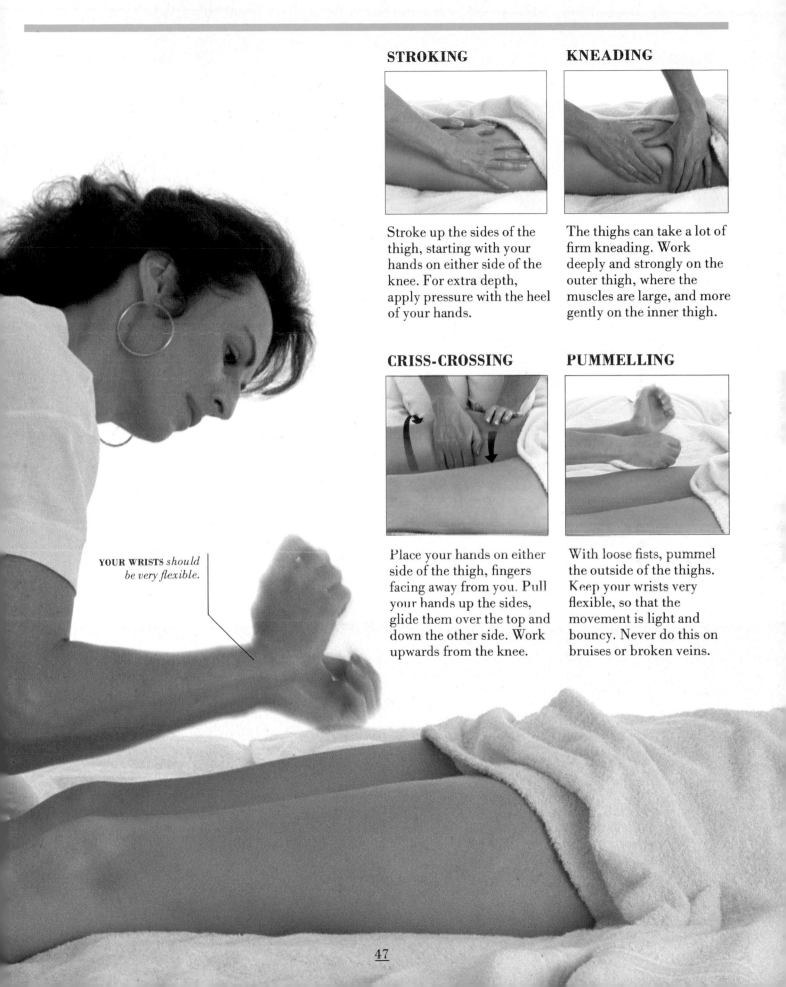

STROKING

Stroke up the sides of the thigh, starting with your hands on either side of the knee. For extra depth, apply pressure with the heel of your hands.

KNEADING

The thighs can take a lot of firm kneading. Work deeply and strongly on the outer thigh, where the muscles are large, and more gently on the inner thigh.

CRISS-CROSSING

Place your hands on either side of the thigh, fingers facing away from you. Pull your hands up the sides, glide them over the top and down the other side. Work upwards from the knee.

PUMMELLING

With loose fists, pummel the outside of the thighs. Keep your wrists very flexible, so that the movement is light and bouncy. Never do this on bruises or broken veins.

YOUR WRISTS *should be very flexible.*

STROKING

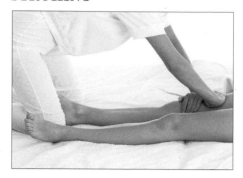

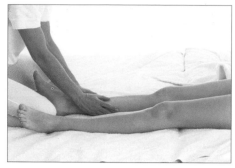

1 Kneel at the feet again and stroke the thigh as before, then stroke the whole leg. Place your hands across the ankle and stroke up the leg, pressing lightly over the bones. Fan your hands out at the top of the thigh.

2 Glide gently back down to the ankle and repeat. Begin with firm, flowing strokes, and gradually slow down. Keep the strokes very rhythmic and make them gentler and gentler until you are barely touching the skin.

THE FINAL TOUCH

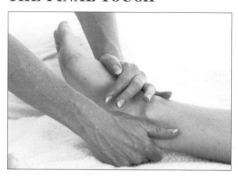

Finish the leg massage in the same way as the foot massage. Hold the foot between your palms, then slide your hands off the end of the foot. Clasp the ankle and stretch the leg gently, then glide your hands off the toes.

PASSIVE MOVEMENTS

Gently flexing the knee and hip is a lovely way of relaxing the leg towards the end of the massage. Kneel beside the hips and, holding the ankle and knee, bend the knee and lift the leg up. Make a large circle with the knee to rotate the hip joint. Circle three times in each direction, making as large a circle as possible, without forcing the joint.

Lean onto the knee to push it gently towards the body. Relax, then repeat. Do this three times, then straighten the leg and lower it gently onto the towel, supporting the knee and ankle.

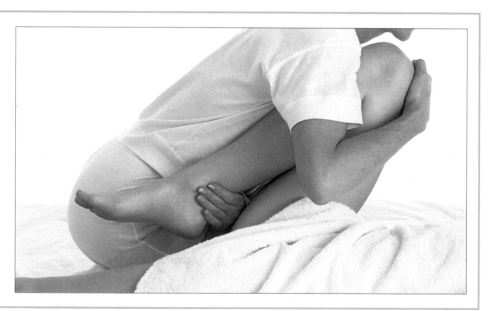

EXTRA MOVEMENTS

You can fit other movements in at any stage of your massage. Experiment to see what your friend enjoys. Knuckling (see page 17) feels very good done on the outside of the thigh. Fast plucking feels marvellous done on the top and outside of the thighs. Work very quickly, grabbing and releasing small bunches of flesh with your thumbs and forefingers. Use your hands alternately, one hand plucking the skin as the other hand releases.

SKIN ROLLING

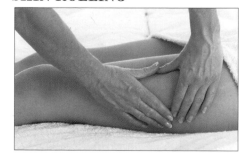

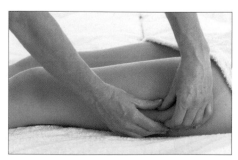

1 This movement improves skin texture and releases tension. Put your hands on the outer thigh, fingers and thumbs together in a triangle.

2 Push your thumbs towards your fingers, rolling the flesh as you do so. Take care not to pinch the skin as your thumbs reach your fingers.

BACK OF THE LEGS

If you are giving a complete body massage, include the back of the legs immediately before or after the back massage. The movements are much the same as for the front of the legs.

1 Stroke the leg from ankle to thigh, pressing gently over the knee.
2 Knead the calf muscles firmly, using both hands.

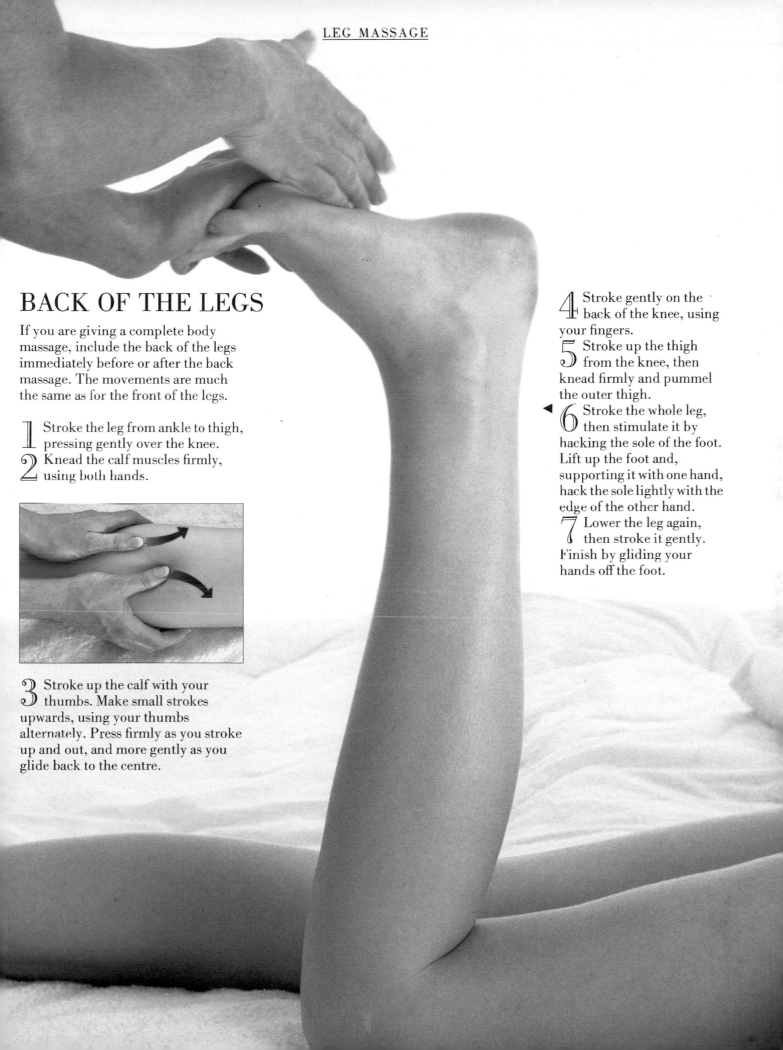

3 Stroke up the calf with your thumbs. Make small strokes upwards, using your thumbs alternately. Press firmly as you stroke up and out, and more gently as you glide back to the centre.

4 Stroke gently on the back of the knee, using your fingers.
5 Stroke up the thigh from the knee, then knead firmly and pummel the outer thigh.
6 Stroke the whole leg, then stimulate it by hacking the sole of the foot. Lift up the foot and, supporting it with one hand, hack the sole lightly with the edge of the other hand.
7 Lower the leg again, then stroke it gently. Finish by gliding your hands off the foot.

HAND MASSAGE

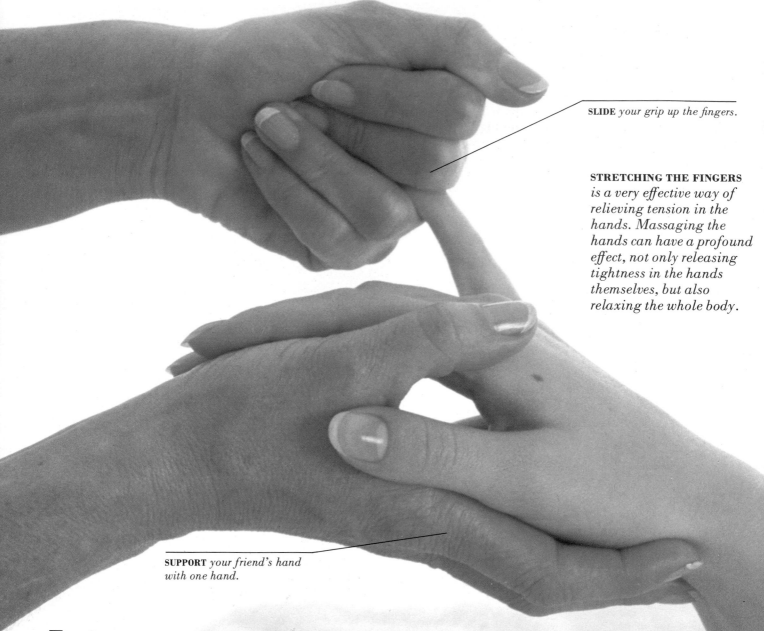

SLIDE *your grip up the fingers.*

STRETCHING THE FINGERS *is a very effective way of relieving tension in the hands. Massaging the hands can have a profound effect, not only releasing tightness in the hands themselves, but also relaxing the whole body.*

SUPPORT *your friend's hand with one hand.*

It always surprises people when they discover the delights of a hand massage. The hands are not normally considered an area of great tension, but as we use our hands in practically everything we do, it is hardly surprising that they sometimes feel stiff and tired. Anyone who constantly uses their hands – anyone, that is, who writes, types, knits, clasps a musical instrument or the handle of a racket, or even those who do massage themselves, will find a regular hand massage of enormous benefit.

The hands are one of the first places to show neglect. As they have very little fat, they become aged and wrinkled very easily. Massaging the hands with cream or oil moisturizes the skin and stimulates the blood supply, keeping the hands soft and smooth.

Hands are easy to reach and, as there is none of the inconvenience of getting undressed, you can give a hand massage anywhere. Everyone is used to having their hands touched, and so people who are slightly nervous of having a massage can be initiated with a hand massage.

I think that to be able to give a hand massage is one of the most useful skills in the world. I have always found it invaluable because, wherever you are, you can always relax and comfort someone with a hand massage.

ANATOMY OF THE HANDS

Our hands are one of the most sensitive parts of the body. They contain thousands of nerve endings, and have proportionally the largest area of the brain to register sensation in the whole body. The fingers are moved by muscles in the forearms, which are attached to the finger bones by long tendons running along the back of the hands.

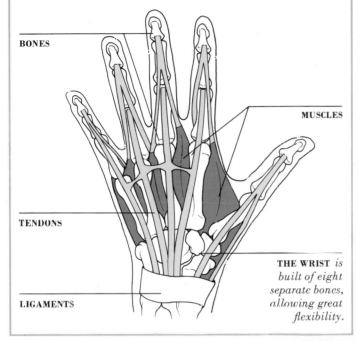

BONES

MUSCLES

TENDONS

THE WRIST *is built of eight separate bones, allowing great flexibility.*

LIGAMENTS

STROKING

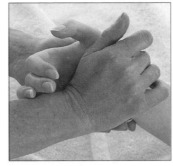

Hold your friend's hand, palm up, in one hand, and stroke the palm with the heel of your other hand. Push down towards the wrist, then glide back.

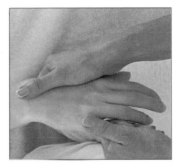

THUMB STROKING

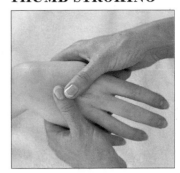

Turn the hand over and support it with your fingers. Stroke the back with your thumbs, making fanning out strokes from the knuckles to the wrist.

STROKE AND STRETCH

Stroke towards the wrist with one hand, moving your fingers up the hand as well as your thumb. Instead of gliding back, pull back firmly to stretch one side of the hand as your other hand strokes up to the wrist.

FINGER MASSAGE

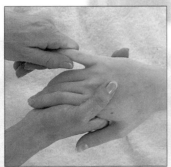
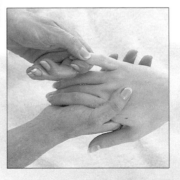
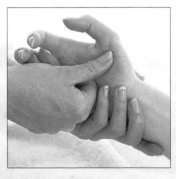

1 Though small and bony, the fingers benefit from a firm massage. Hold your friend's hand palm down in one hand and use the other to work on each finger separately. Stroke from the tip to the knuckle, then squeeze all over the finger.

2 Do circular pressures round each joint with your thumb, then rotate the finger twice in each direction. Finally, make your hand into a fist and grip the finger between two of your fingers (see main picture opposite). Stretch it gently to ease the joints, but don't jerk it.

3 Change hands when you reach the thumb and massage it deeply and thoroughly. Strong, firm pressure usually feels good here; gentle pressure can be irritating. Turn the hand over to do firm circular pressures all over the muscular area at the base of the thumb.

STROKING BETWEEN THE TENDONS

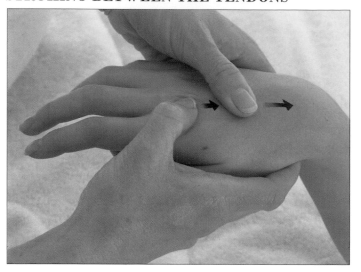

Turn the hand over and support it with your fingers. Stroke with your thumbs in the furrows between the tendons, starting between the knuckles and stroking towards the wrist, one thumb following the other. Do this a few times in each furrow, then turn the hand over and stroke the palm firmly with the heel of your hand, as you did at the start.

KNUCKLING

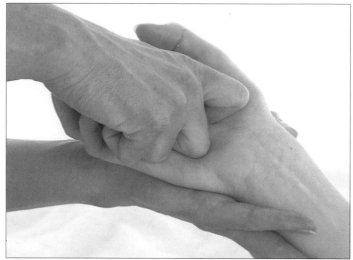

Make a fist with one hand and support your friend's hand, palm up, with your other hand. Move your fist all over the palm, making small, rippling, circular movements with your knuckles. Vary the pressure from deep to gentle – both feel marvellous. This movement is also good for your hands, increasing their flexibility and coordination.

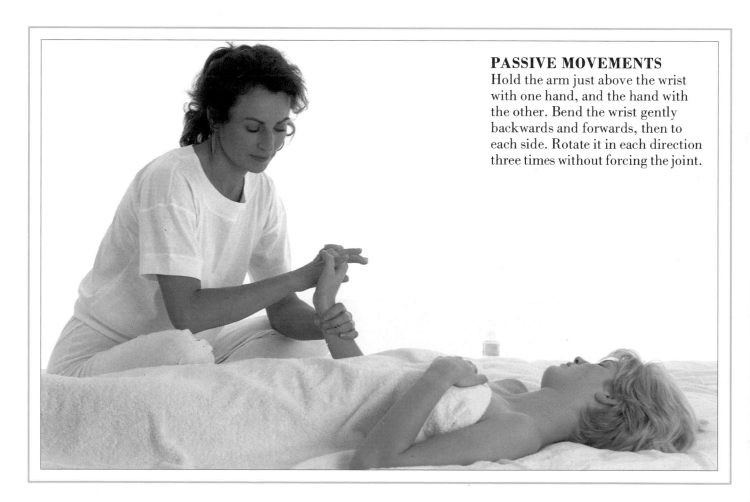

PASSIVE MOVEMENTS
Hold the arm just above the wrist with one hand, and the hand with the other. Bend the wrist gently backwards and forwards, then to each side. Rotate it in each direction three times without forcing the joint.

STRETCHING THE HAND

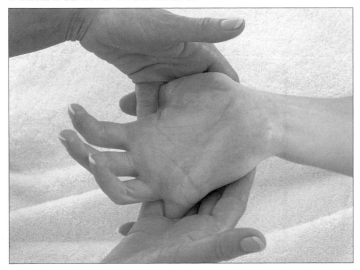

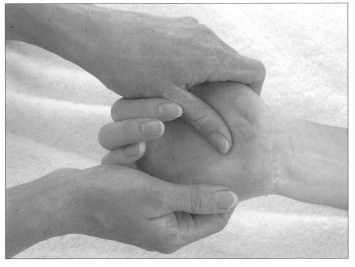

1 With your hands palm up, interlock your little fingers with your friend's hand, one with her little finger, one with her thumb. Bring your other fingers underneath the hand to support it, then open the hand to stretch the palm. This counteracts our normal clutching movements and helps to release tension from the hands.

2 Keep your little fingers interlocked with your friend's hand, and continue to stretch the palm. Bring your thumbs round onto the palm and stroke it all over with fanning out movements. Then, using only one thumb, make small circular pressures all over the palm. It can be tense anywhere, and firm pressure feels very good.

WRIST MASSAGE

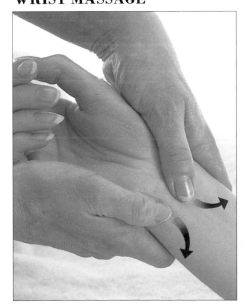

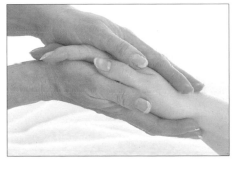

THE FINAL TOUCH

1 ◀Stroke the whole hand, then turn it over and sandwich it between your palms. Press them together firmly for a couple of seconds.

2 ▼Release the pressure and slide your hands slowly off the fingers. The hand should now be completely relaxed. Repeat this a couple of times.

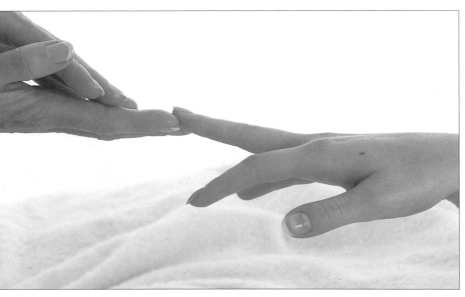

Support the hand with your fingers and stroke all round the wrist with your thumbs. Start on the inside of the wrist and stroke towards the arm and out to the sides. Work with both thumbs together and then alternately. Turn the hand over and work in the same way on the other side, pushing firmly towards the body and gliding back.

ARM MASSAGE

As the arms are so small in comparison with the rest of the body, many people learning massage want to leave them out altogether, as they seem insignificant. They are not. Headaches, neck pain, and aching shoulders or tired hands can all be caused by tension in the arms. Massaging the arms helps the arms and shoulders to relax, and can alleviate many of these problems.

You may find the arm a little awkward to massage at first, because it is small and bony. Do not be deterred by its size: the muscles are usually strong and your massage can be deep and firm. The techniques are almost exactly the same as those used on the legs, and with a little practice you will find arm massage easy and rewarding. Kneel beside your friend to give the massage.

STROKING

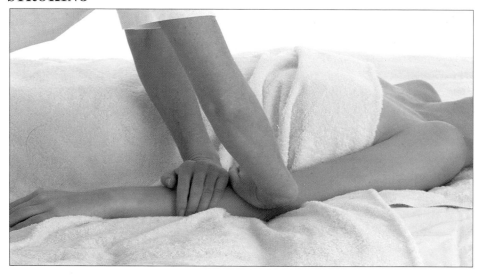

1 Rest your friend's arm, palm down, on the towel and place your hands across her wrist, with the little finger of one next to the thumb of the other. Stroke firmly up the arm with your hands slightly cupped so that the pressure is deep on the muscle, but light over the bones.

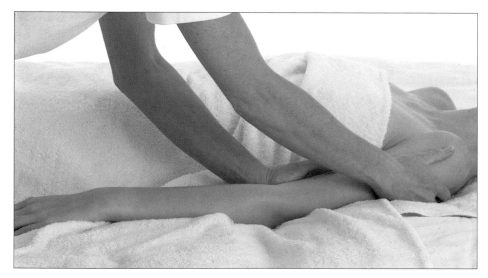

2 When you reach the top of the arm, open your hands out and stroke round the shoulder. Make sure that you reach right round the top of the shoulder with one hand, then glide your hands lightly down the sides of the arms to your friend's wrist, ready to start again. Repeat about six times.

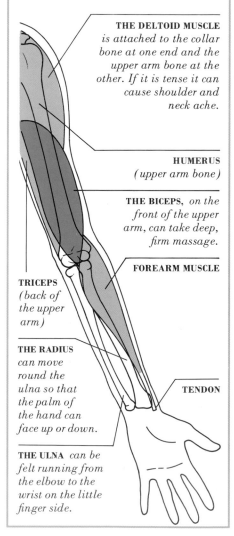

ANATOMY OF THE ARM
The bones of the arms and hands are much more delicate than those of the legs and feet, but the general arrangement is very similar. The two bones in the forearm are approximately the same size, and can be felt clearly because there is not much muscle lying over them.

THE DELTOID MUSCLE *is attached to the collar bone at one end and the upper arm bone at the other. If it is tense it can cause shoulder and neck ache.*

HUMERUS *(upper arm bone)*

THE BICEPS, *on the front of the upper arm, can take deep, firm massage.*

FOREARM MUSCLE

TRICEPS *(back of the upper arm)*

THE RADIUS *can move round the ulna so that the palm of the hand can face up or down.*

TENDON

THE ULNA *can be felt running from the elbow to the wrist on the little finger side.*

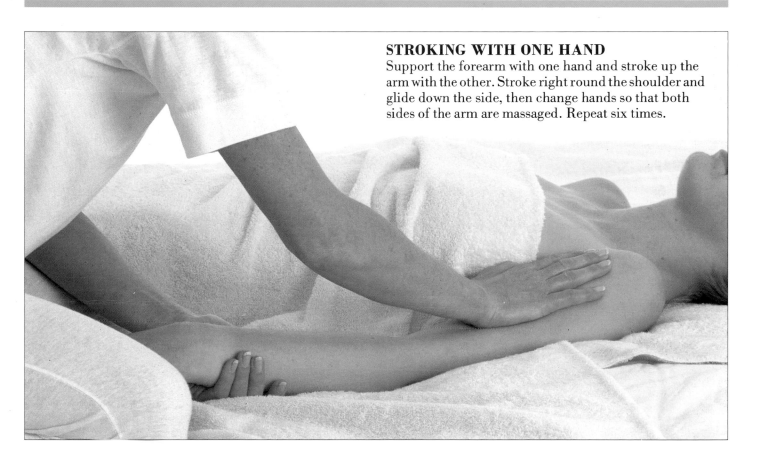

STROKING WITH ONE HAND
Support the forearm with one hand and stroke up the arm with the other. Stroke right round the shoulder and glide down the side, then change hands so that both sides of the arm are massaged. Repeat six times.

DRAINING THE FOREARM

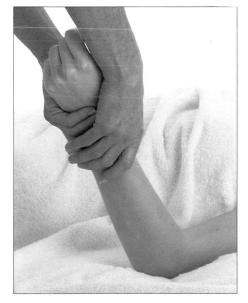

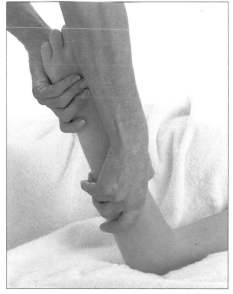

FAN STROKING

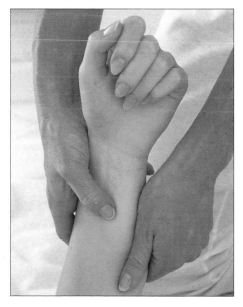

1 This movement improves drainage of waste products from the veins of the forearm. Lift up your friend's forearm, supporting the wrist and leaving the elbow on the towel. Clasp your hands round her wrist, with your thumbs on the inside of the wrist.

2 Slide one hand down to the elbow, pressing with your thumb but not your fingers. When you reach the elbow, glide lightly back to the wrist. As the first hand returns to the wrist, stroke down with the other hand. Repeat three or four times.

With your hands in the same position, make fanning out strokes with your thumbs on the inside of the wrist. Use your thumbs alternately, one stroking firmly down and out as the other glides back. Gradually lengthen the strokes until you cover the whole forearm.

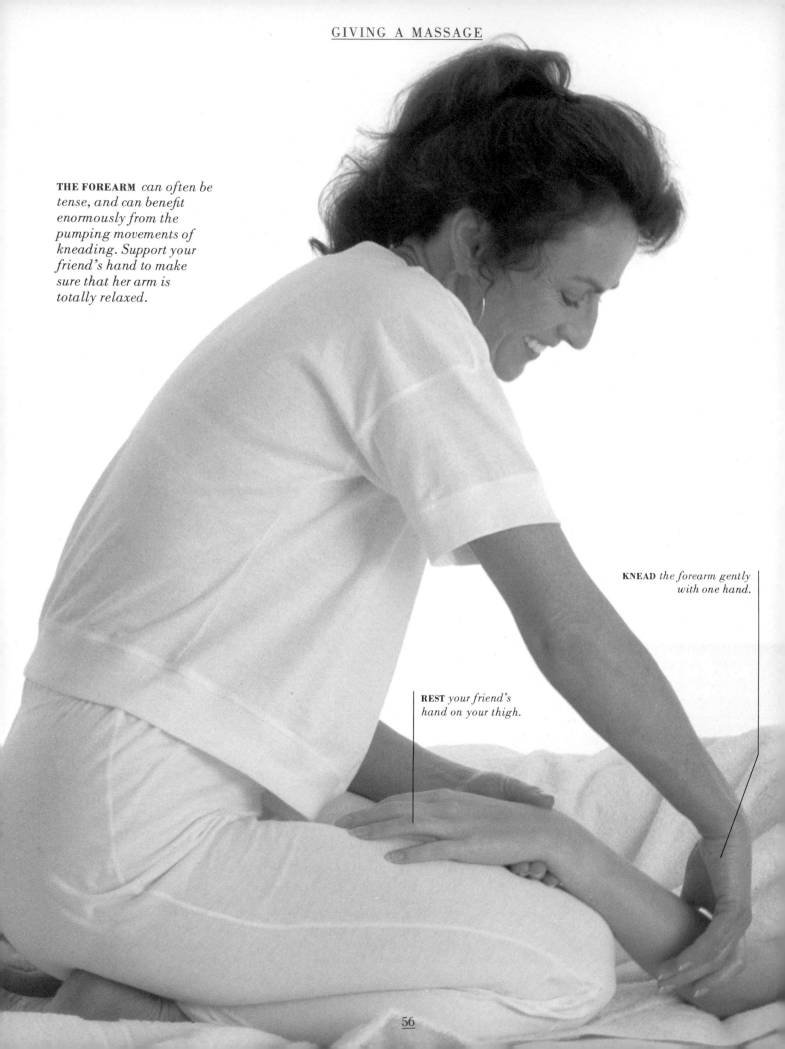

THE FOREARM *can often be tense, and can benefit enormously from the pumping movements of kneading. Support your friend's hand to make sure that her arm is totally relaxed.*

KNEAD *the forearm gently with one hand.*

REST *your friend's hand on your thigh.*

KNEADING

1 ► Knead the forearm gently with one hand, working from the wrist to the elbow, then glide your hand down to start again. Repeat a couple of times, then change hands to knead the other side.

2 ▼ Knead the same area with both hands, resting your friend's hand on your thigh or your knee.

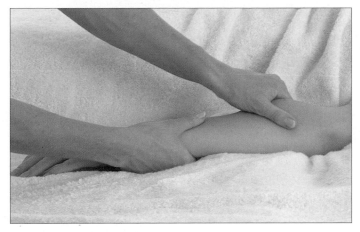

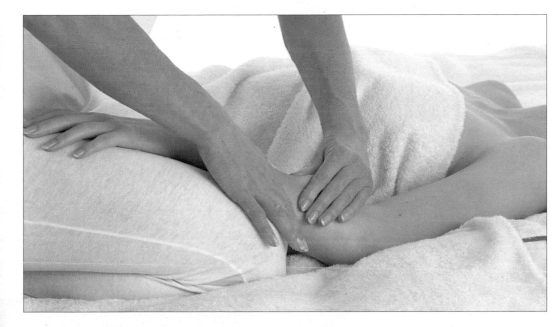

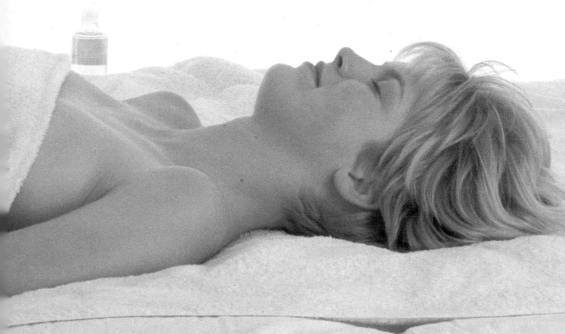

ELBOW MASSAGE

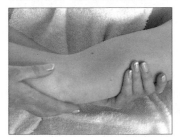

1 Leave her hand on your thigh, support the arm with one hand, and stroke her elbow with the other.

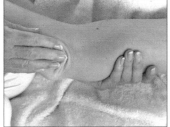

2 Stroke smoothly in a circle all round the elbow, using just the tips of your fingers.

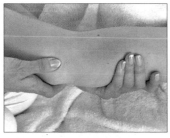

3 With your fingers on one side and your thumb on the other, do circular pressures all over the elbow. Be thorough: work into all the nooks and crannies. Elbows tend to be neglected, and massage here feels surprisingly good. Use plenty of oil: they are often dry, and will soak it up. Finish by stroking again to soothe the area.

CIRCLE STROKING THE UPPER ARM

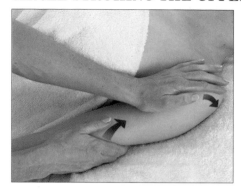

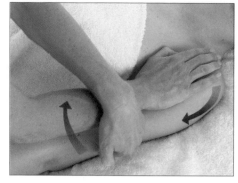

1 Stroke from the elbow upwards with one hand, moulding it to the shape of the arm. When you reach the shoulder, press it down gently and begin stroking with your other hand.

2 Glide your first hand round the shoulder and down the outside of the arm. Lift it away as your second hand strokes round the shoulder, and start again at the elbow.

KNEADING

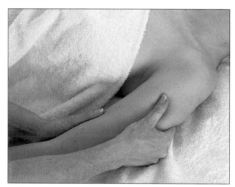

Support the arm with one hand and knead the upper arm with the other. Work up the arm on both sides. Or rest the arm on the towel and knead with one hand on either side of the arm.

If the arm is large enough, you can work with both hands together on one side. Knead firmly up the arm from the elbow, wringing and squeezing the flesh without hurting or pinching.

FEATHER STROKING

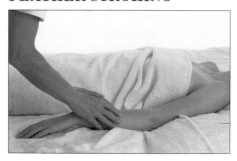

Stroke down the whole arm with both hands together, gradually becoming lighter and lighter until you are barely touching the skin.

FINAL TOUCH

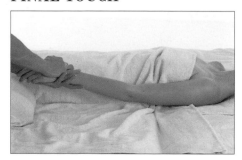

Clasp the wrist and lean back to stretch the arm gently. Finish by holding the hand and then gliding your hands very slowly off the fingers.

PASSIVE MOVEMENTS

The whole arm should be limp and relaxed after the massage. This is a good time to loosen the shoulder joints thoroughly with some gentle passive movements. Hold your friend's wrist with one hand and lift her arm up over her head. Stretch it as far as it will comfortably go, and slide your other hand down to her hip to give a lovely long stretch. Then bring her arm down to her side again. Hold her hand in both of your hands and, with her arm outstretched, shake the whole arm gently up and down. Finish with a gentle pull.

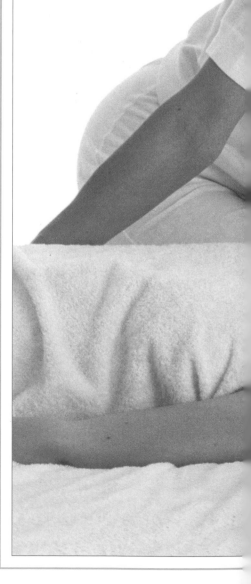

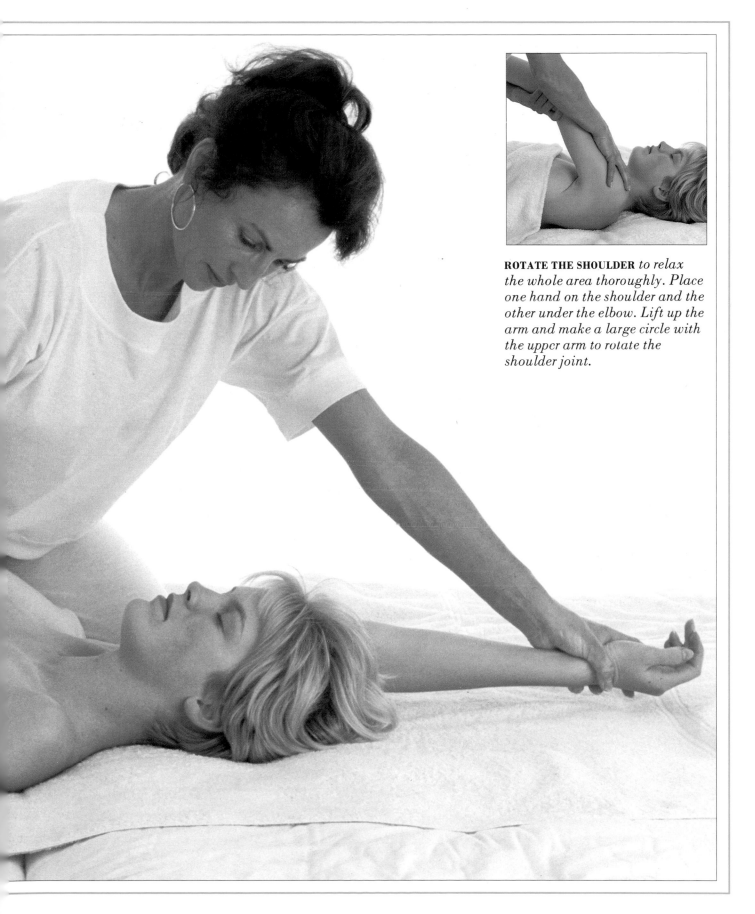

ROTATE THE SHOULDER *to relax the whole area thoroughly. Place one hand on the shoulder and the other under the elbow. Lift up the arm and make a large circle with the upper arm to rotate the shoulder joint.*

ABDOMEN MASSAGE

At first some people are a little apprehensive of having their abdomen massaged. I think this is because they carry their tension there, and to expose the abdomen makes them feel vulnerable. But anyone who experiences the delights of a good abdomen massage will be converted.

I teach a very gentle, relaxing abdomen massage, which calms the nerves and stimulates the digestive system. If you suffer from stomach aches, whether caused by tension, indigestion or a bad period, this massage can soothe them away. The calming, relaxing strokes can also relieve constipation. Abdomen massage is useful to weight-watchers: by making them aware of the area, it helps them to keep to a diet far more

conscientiously, and by stimulating the circulation it improves skin texture.

Some people advise one not to give an abdomen massage to pregnant women, but I have found that they benefit greatly from a very gentle massage on the abdomen: it soothes both the mother and the baby. For details on how to massage during pregnancy, see pages 98 to 101.

When you massage the abdomen, all your movements should be gentle and sensitive. Kneel beside the waist and place a pillow under your friend's knees to help relax the back and stomach muscles. The basic massage takes five to ten minutes, but you can make it last as long as you like by repeating the movements.

STROKING

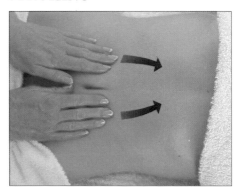

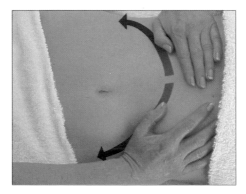

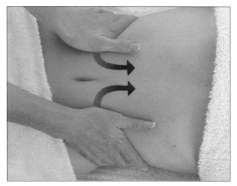

1 Face towards the head and place your hands side by side on the lower abdomen, fingers pointing towards the head. Stroke slowly up to the ribs, keeping the pressure even.

2 When you reach the ribs, pull your hands out to the sides and glide them down. Mould your hands to the curves of the body, making sure you don't leave any bits unstroked.

3 Pull your hands firmly up and in at the sides of the waist, then swivel round to start again. Keep the movement flowing and continuous, and repeat at least six times.

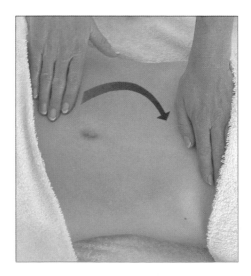

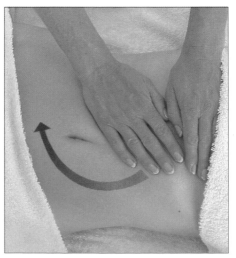

CIRCLING THE NAVEL

1 ◄◄Turn to face across the body, and put your left hand on the lower ribs. Start with your right hand below the navel and stroke gently in a wide curve up towards your left hand, keeping the pressure smooth and light.

2 ◄Continue stroking with your right hand in a circle round the navel. Always stroke in a clockwise direction when massaging the abdomen. This simple movement is extremely comforting, so repeat it at any time in the massage if you need to spread extra oil.

CIRCLE STROKING

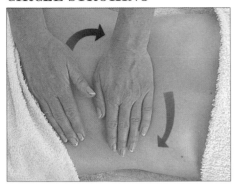

1 As for the previous movement, stroke clockwise round the abdomen, but this time use both hands. Place your hands on the abdomen and begin stroking round in a circle, one hand following the other.

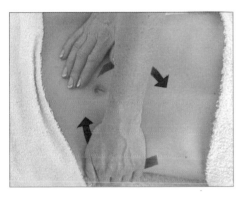

2 Glide your left hand round the far side of the waist, while your right hand strokes up the abdomen. Keep the pressure gentle as you glide down the side and firmer as you pull in at the waist and stroke up the abdomen.

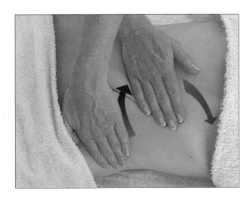

3 Sweep your left hand up the side of the waist and your right hand across the abdomen. Your arms cross as you stroke round in a circle.

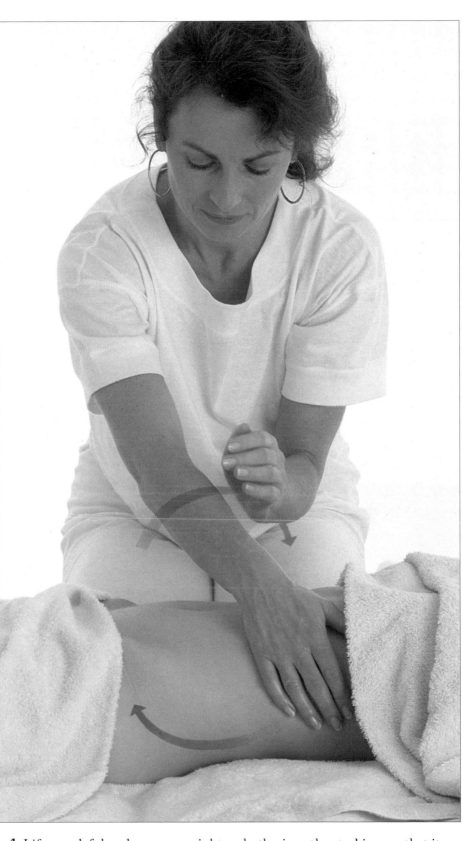

4 Lift your left hand over your right arm and place it gently on the abdomen to start again. Keep the return movement as smooth and rhythmic as the stroking, so that it feels like one continuous circle. This soothing movement can relieve a stomach ache.

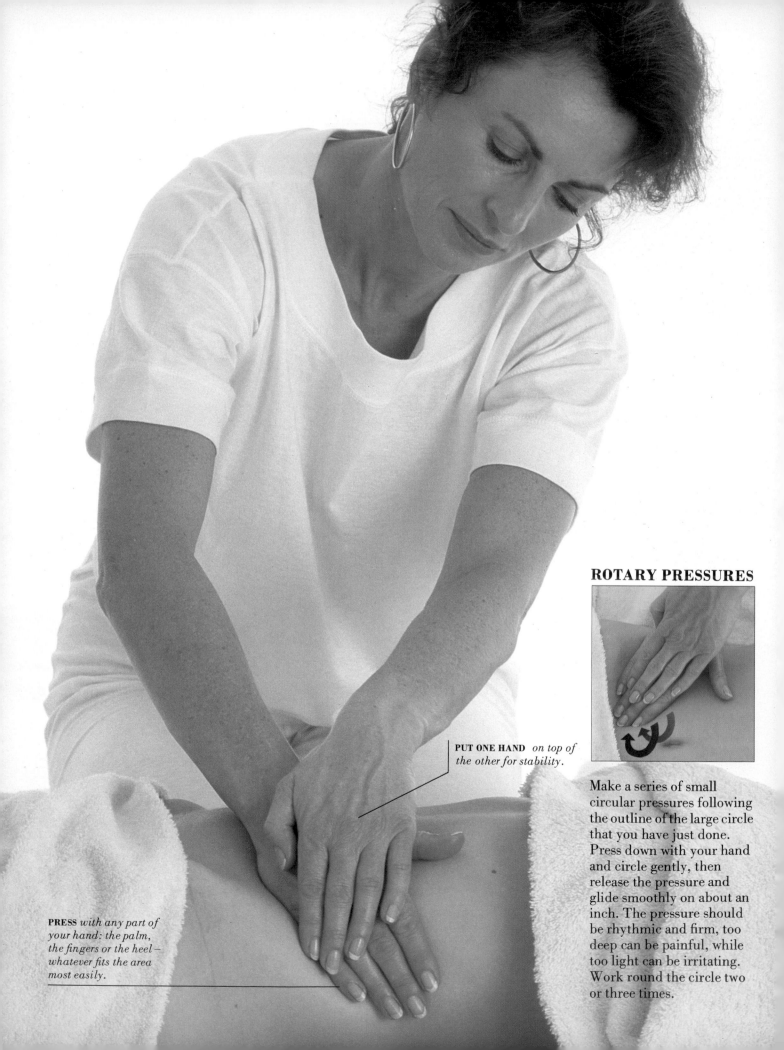

ROTARY PRESSURES

PUT ONE HAND *on top of
the other for stability.*

Make a series of small
circular pressures following
the outline of the large circle
that you have just done.
Press down with your hand
and circle gently, then
release the pressure and
glide smoothly on about an
inch. The pressure should
be rhythmic and firm, too
deep can be painful, while
too light can be irritating.
Work round the circle two
or three times.

PRESS *with any part of
your hand: the palm,
the fingers or the heel —
whatever fits the area
most easily.*

KNEADING

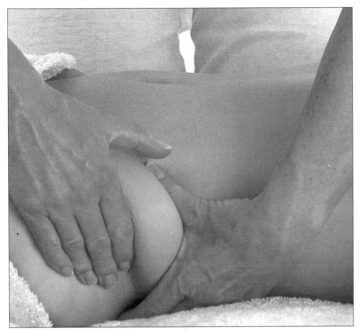

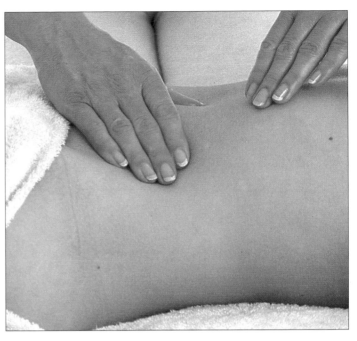

1 Knead the whole area, starting with the hip on the far side of the body. With your hands facing each other and your elbows out, alternately squeeze and release the flesh – there is often a good handful to get hold of. Work thoroughly over the whole hip: your kneading can be deep and stimulating.

2 Work up the side of the waist and gently across the abdomen. Depending on your friend's size, you may find it easier to use just your fingers and thumbs rather than your whole hands. Lift, press and squeeze the flesh without pinching. Do several rows of light kneading across the abdomen, then knead the side and hip nearest you.

SIDE STROKING

CRISS-CROSSING

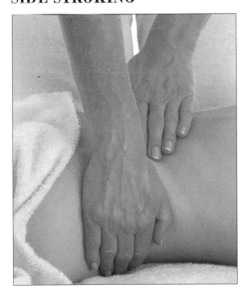

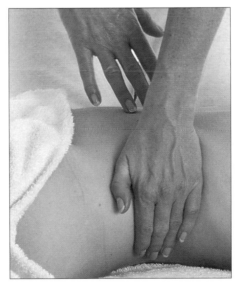

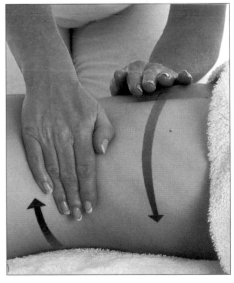

1 This soothing stroke is very calming after the kneading. With relaxed hands, stroke slowly up the side of the waist. One hand follows the other as you stroke rhythmically and lazily in towards the navel.

2 Lift the first hand off as you reach the navel and repeat. When working on the side nearest you, either lean down and push up with your hands, or twist round so that you can still pull up with your hands.

Start with your hands on either side of the waist, then pull up the sides and glide across the abdomen. Make a definite contrast between pulling up firmly and stroking across very gently. Do this at least six times.

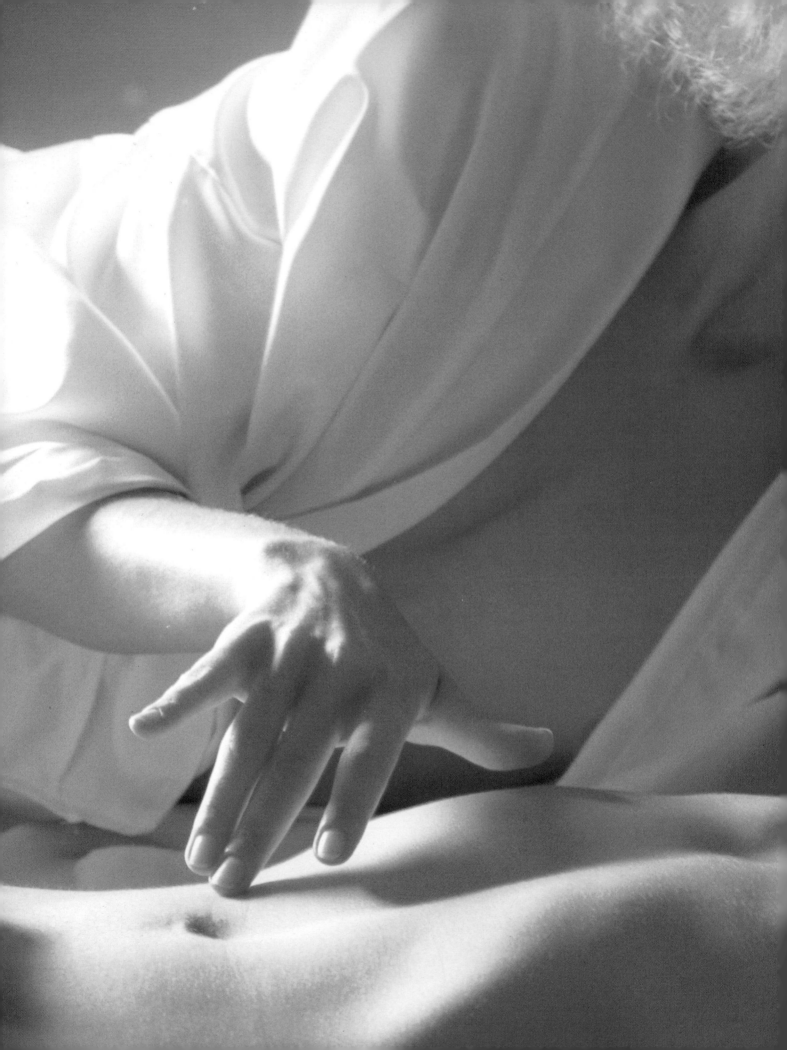

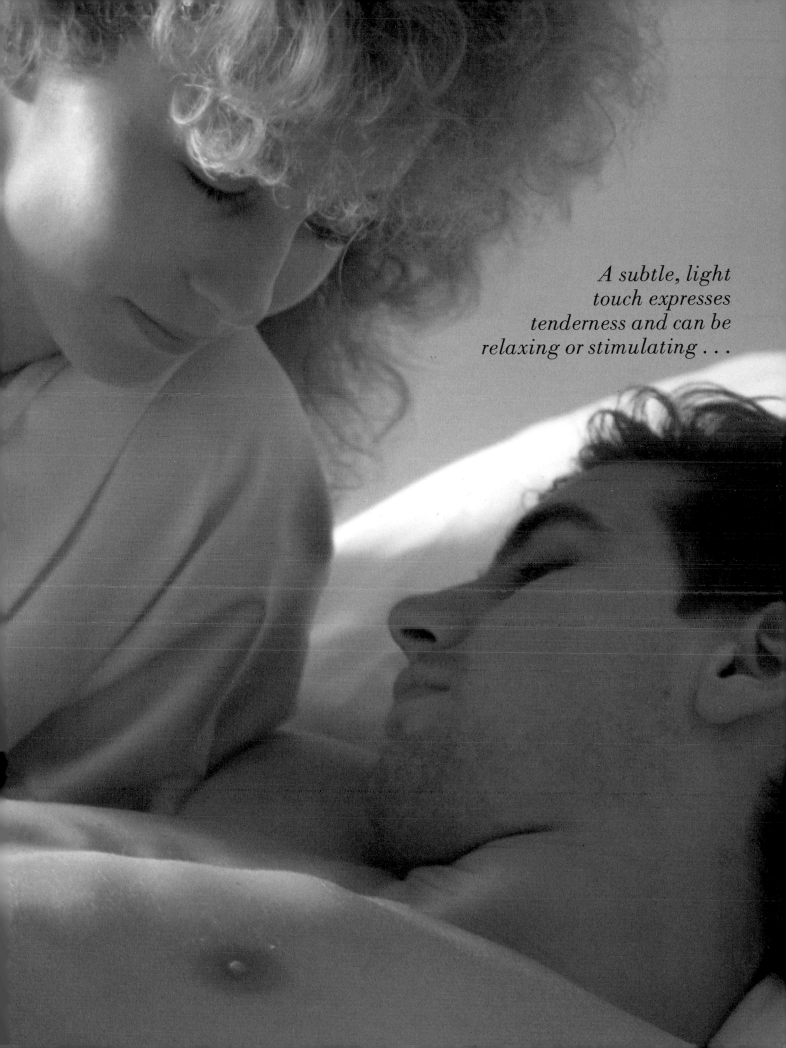

A subtle, light touch expresses tenderness and can be relaxing or stimulating . . .

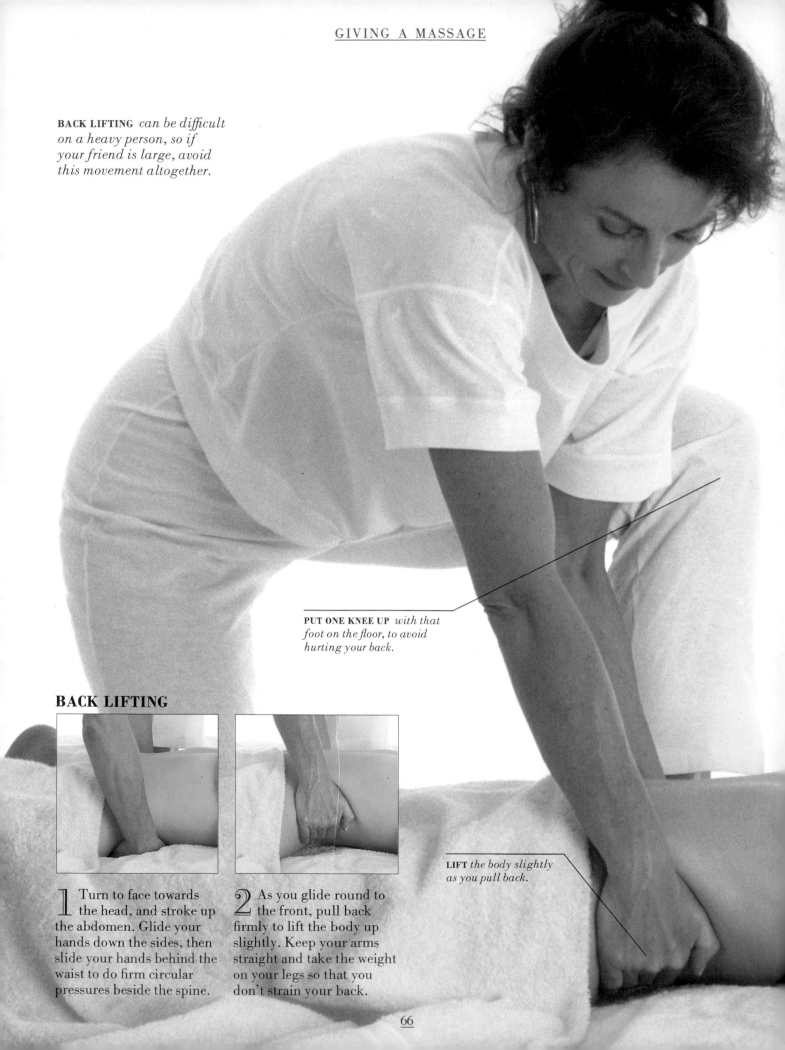

BACK LIFTING *can be difficult on a heavy person, so if your friend is large, avoid this movement altogether.*

PUT ONE KNEE UP *with that foot on the floor, to avoid hurting your back.*

BACK LIFTING

LIFT *the body slightly as you pull back.*

1 Turn to face towards the head, and stroke up the abdomen. Glide your hands down the sides, then slide your hands behind the waist to do firm circular pressures beside the spine.

2 As you glide round to the front, pull back firmly to lift the body up slightly. Keep your arms straight and take the weight on your legs so that you don't strain your back.

INDIAN FLOWER SELLER

I learnt this slow, deep movement from a flower seller in India, who used it to relieve my terrible stomach ache. Never use this on a pregnant woman. Place one hand on top of the other, fingers just below the navel, and stroke up infinitely slowly. Maintain a deep pressure until you pass the navel, then release the pressure and glide back.

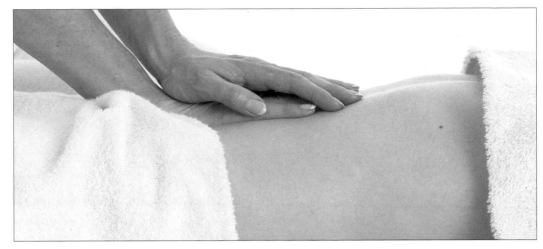

FEATHER STROKING

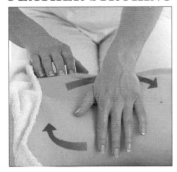 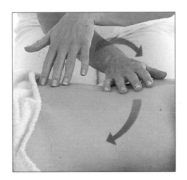

1 You are nearing the end of the massage, so do lots of stroking. Repeat the initial stroking, then turn to face across the body and flow smoothly into the circle stroking.

2 Stroke clockwise in a circle, one hand following the other. Gradually stroke more and more softly until you are barely touching the skin. Continue for as long as you like.

THE FINAL TOUCH

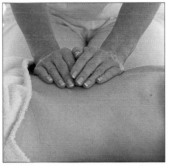 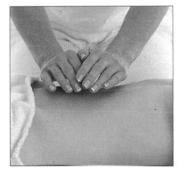

1 This simple technique has a dramatic effect, leaving your friend feeling relaxed and light. Cup your hands over the navel to trap some air underneath. Hold them still for a few seconds and feel heat gathering. Ease the warmth into the body by slightly flattening your hands.

2 Relax your hands and lift them very, very slowly away from the body. You must not hurry this movement: take your time. As your hands leave the body, the person being massaged often feels a floating sensation, as if you are drawing out tension and lifting the body.

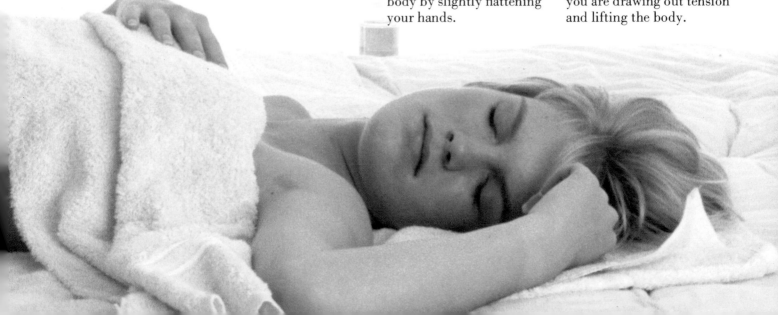

CHEST AND NECK MASSAGE

I am always surprised at how many people carry tension in their chests. Bad posture and rounded shoulders make the chest muscles very tense. Sitting cramped over a desk, hunching over the steering wheel of a car, even sports such as horse riding and golf, and illnesses such as asthma, can all put a strain on these muscles. The chest muscles shorten and contract, and the muscles in the upper back become overstretched. This makes the spine constantly rounded, so that the neck juts forwards and the head pokes up, causing tight, inflexible muscles in the neck and all round the shoulders.

Massage can help to stretch and relax the chest muscles, thus alleviating aching in the upper back and neck. Working on the muscles between the ribs can help to straighten out the shoulders.

The ideal time to do a chest massage is before you massage the face, but it also fits in well after one arm massage and before the other, or after the stomach or back massage.

Your friend should lie on his back, and you should kneel behind his head. Put a small cushion or a thick book (a telephone directory is ideal) under his head so that his neck is perfectly relaxed. This is a good position for working on the shoulders, and since it is difficult to relax the chest and neck unless the shoulders are relaxed too, I always include them in the massage when I am working on this area.

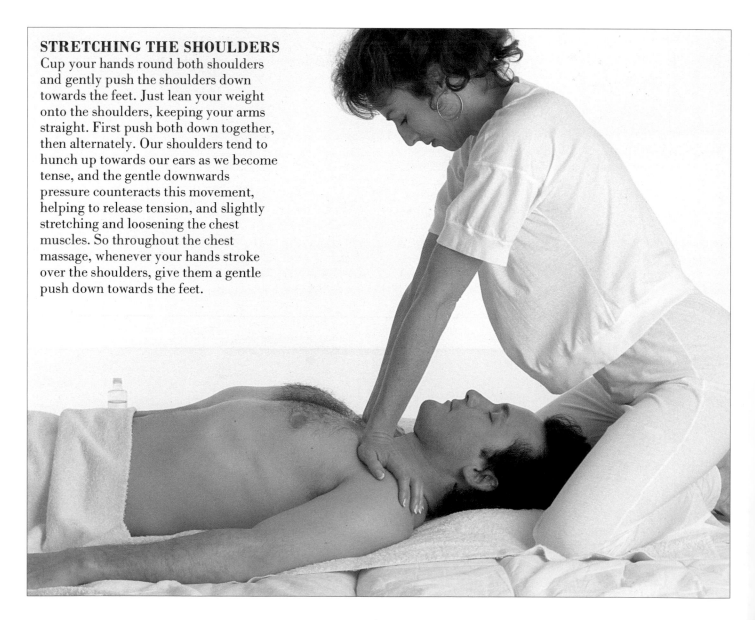

STRETCHING THE SHOULDERS
Cup your hands round both shoulders and gently push the shoulders down towards the feet. Just lean your weight onto the shoulders, keeping your arms straight. First push both down together, then alternately. Our shoulders tend to hunch up towards our ears as we become tense, and the gentle downwards pressure counteracts this movement, helping to release tension, and slightly stretching and loosening the chest muscles. So throughout the chest massage, whenever your hands stroke over the shoulders, give them a gentle push down towards the feet.

STROKING

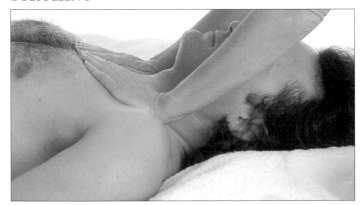

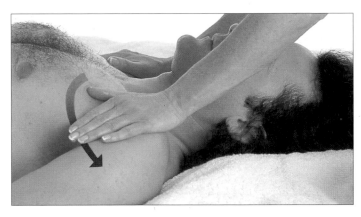

1 Spread the oil by stroking the whole area. Try to make the movement feel firm and flowing. Start with your hands next to each other, just below the collar-bones at the base of the neck.

2 Stroke down the chest to the breast, keeping the pressure smooth but firm. Then fan your hands out and, keeping them relaxed, glide out across the chest towards the shoulders.

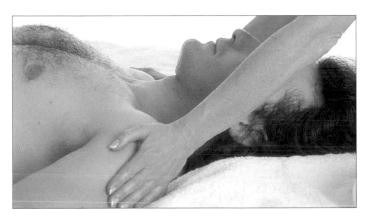

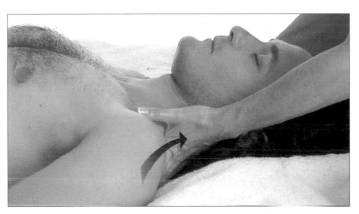

3 Make sure your hands mould to the contours of the body as you stroke over the shoulders. Cup them over the shoulders and gently press the shoulders towards the feet or down onto the floor.

4 Swing your fingers round to the back of the shoulders and stroke behind the shoulders and up the back of the neck. Then glide your hands down the sides of the neck to the collar-bones. Repeat at least four times.

KNUCKLING

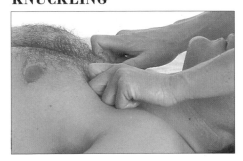

Make your hands into fists and ripple your fingers round to make small circular movements with your knuckles. Work all over the chest, then behind the shoulders and all round the base of the neck.

DEEP PRESSURES

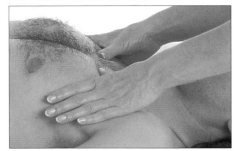

Do a series of thumb pressures on the muscles between the ribs. Start in the middle and work in lines out towards the shoulders. Pressures in this area can be painful, so the depth depends on your friend's reaction.

KNEADING

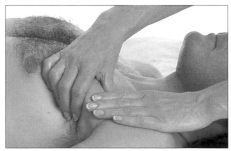

Knead the fleshy area in front of the armpit, picking up and squeezing the muscle with alternate hands. Work with both hands on one side, then on the other side. This will release tension in the chest, arms and back.

ALTERNATE STROKING

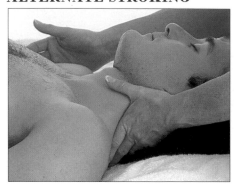

With one hand on each side of the neck, stroke with alternate hands from the shoulders to the base of the skull. Sway from side to side to make the stroke large and even as you gently push the head from side to side.

SIDE STROKING

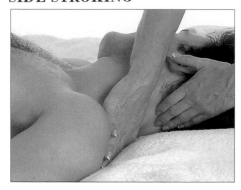

1 Now use both hands on one side. Lean slightly towards the side you are working on, and stroke with one hand from the shoulder up the neck to the base of the skull. As it reaches the ear, follow it with the other hand.

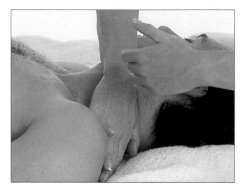

2 Lift the first hand off and return it to the shoulder as the second hand strokes up the neck. Keep the return movement smooth, so that the whole sequence feels flowing. Repeat several times on one side, then change sides.

SIDE STRETCH

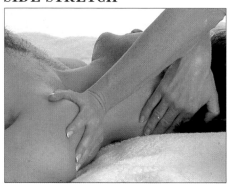

Cup one hand over one shoulder, and the other round the base of the skull on the same side. Gently push the shoulder down and pull the head without jerking the neck, to stretch the neck. Repeat on the other side.

PRESSURES

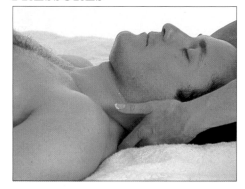

1 With the two middle fingers of each hand, make small, firm, circular pressures on either side of the spine. Work up the neck, then press into the hollow at the top of the spine and the indentations on either side.

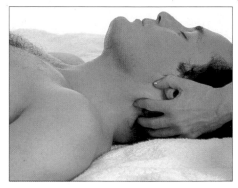

2 Make circular pressures all over the base of the skull. Press firmly, but with care: the muscles here are frequently taut and tense, and these pressures, which stimulate blood flow, can unknot the tension.

PASSIVE MOVEMENTS

1 Tension all down the back and up to the top of the head can be relieved by stretching the neck. Apply the stretch very gradually and smoothly, never jerk or pull suddenly. Cup your hands round the base of the skull and, without lifting the head up, lean back slowly, using your body weight to give a gentle stretch to the neck. Repeat two or three times.

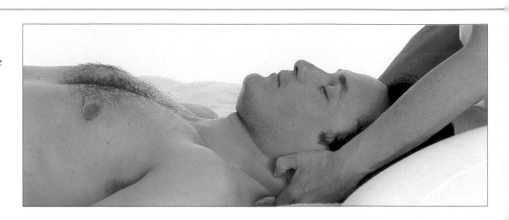

EXTRA MOVEMENT

This is a lovely way of opening the chest and relaxing the shoulders and the whole back. Ask your friend to lift up slightly, then slide your hands as far under his back as you can reach. Slowly pull up the back, taking your friend's weight in your hands. Use your own body weight to stretch the spine slowly. If your friend is much heavier than you, this may be a little difficult and even on a small person, you must use your body properly to avoid straining your back.

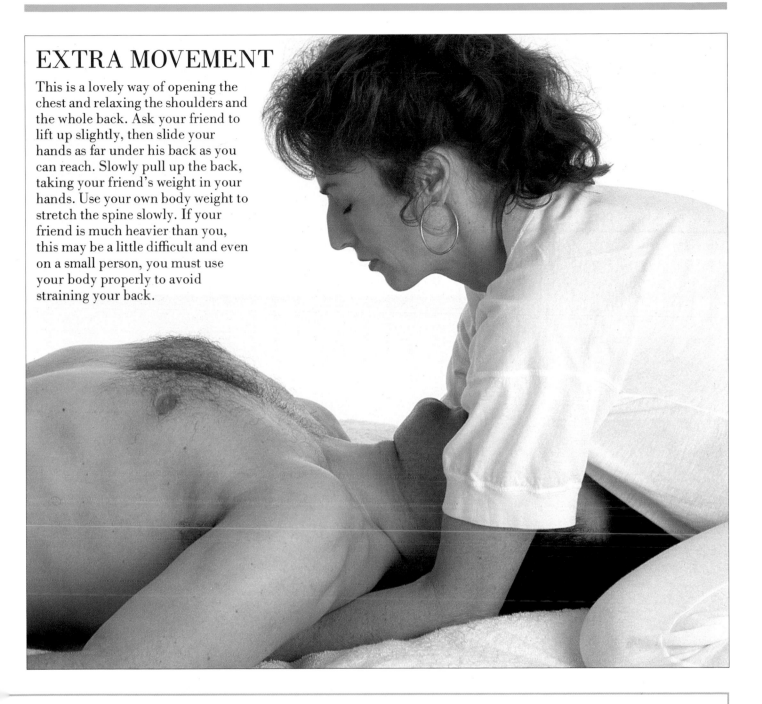

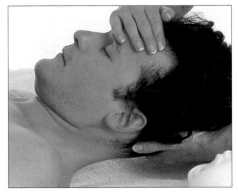

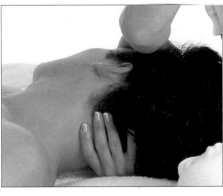

2 ◄◄ Cup one hand round the back of the head and place the other on the forehead. Lift the head so that the chin drops forwards, then lower the head, letting your hand take its weight. Repeat until the head moves freely.

3 ◄ With your hands in the same position, slowly turn the head from side to side, supporting it all the time. It should move freely.

FACE MASSAGE

A good face massage can soothe away anxiety, headaches and exhaustion, to replace them with a feeling of serenity and well-being. It also benefits appearance, leaving people looking and feeling years younger. By improving the circulation, it gives a healthy and vibrant glow to the complexion. By relaxing taut muscles, it rids the face of that tired, pinched expression. So dramatic is its effect, that one client opted for a regular face massage instead of having a face lift.

Men don't usually think of having a face massage, though they can benefit just as much as women. Several foreign statesmen, who had had regular massage all their lives, had never had a face massage until they came to me. Now they always have their faces included in a massage. I think everyone should do the same – it is such a simple way of removing worry and tension, even if only temporarily.

To give a good face massage, your hands must be relaxed, and your movements should feel flowing and confident. This needs experience, so either practise on your own face first, or try out the movements on your knee.

Kneel behind your friend's head and use a fine face oil or an enriched face cream. Be sure to use enough lubrication to avoid dragging the skin. Check that your hands are clean, with no rough skin and that your nails aren't so long that they scratch the face. Ask your friend to remove contact lenses if he wears them. Use the initial stroking sequence throughout the massage to give continuity and link your movements from area to area.

STROKING

1 ▶ This rhythmic stroke covers the entire face and spreads the oil. It should feel flowing and smooth, and initiates your friend to the massage. Start with your hands at the base of the neck, then sweep them up to the chin, using the whole surface of your hands. Pause for a moment.

2 ▶▶ Stroke out under the jaw to the ears, moulding your hands to the contours of the face. Pause for a moment with your palms resting over the ears, then glide your hands back down under the chin.

3 ▶ Stroke with your fingertips from the chin, round the mouth, to the nostrils (be careful not to block them). Continue stroking up the sides of the nose, pause just below the eyes, then glide out gently under the cheek-bones and up to the temples, then back down to the chin.

4 ▶▶ Stroke up the front of the face again, but this time continue up to the bridge of the nose. Pause, then stroke out across the forehead to the temples. Pause and press, then glide down to the chin. Do the whole sequence at least four times.

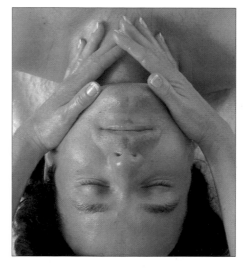
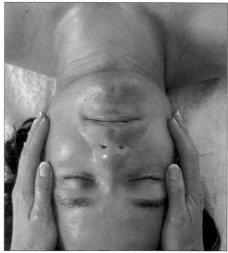
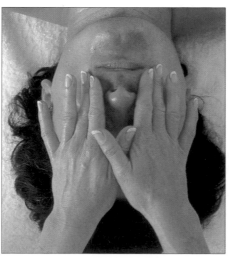
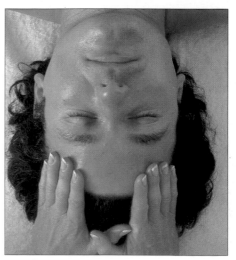

CUPPING THE FACE

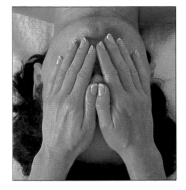

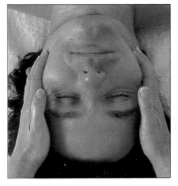

1 Cup your hands over the face, with the palms on the forehead and the fingers over the mouth. Hold them there for a moment.

2 Press down very gently, then release the pressure and draw your hands out to the sides. Pause here for a moment, then repeat.

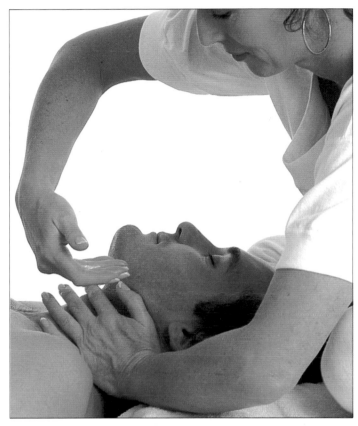

NECK STROKING▶

Now work with both hands on one side. Stroke with one hand firmly up the neck from the shoulder to the ear, then lift it away and start stroking with the other hand on the same side. Repeat about six times on each side.

PAT UNDER THE JAW

Continue stimulating the jawline by patting and slapping under the chin. Use the ring and middle fingers of each hand to slap under the jawline. It is a bouncy percussion movement, which should stimulate but not sting. Afterwards, soothe the area by stroking gently.

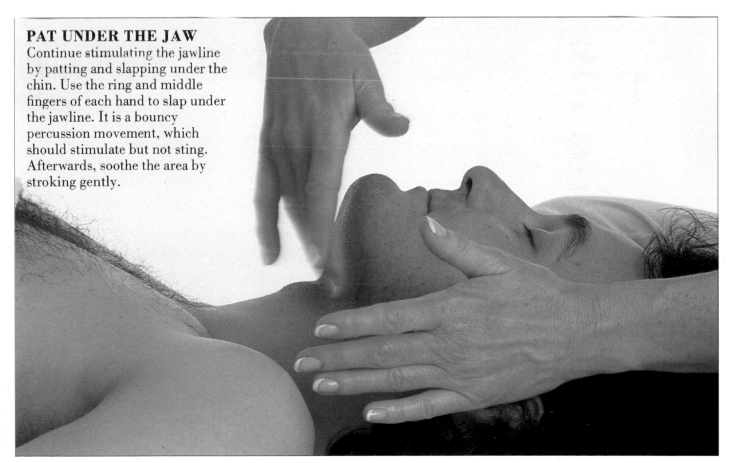

MASSAGING THE CHEEKS

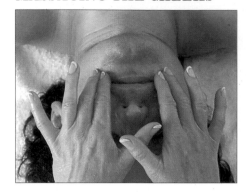 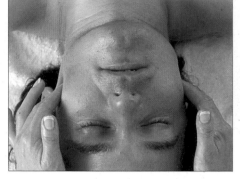 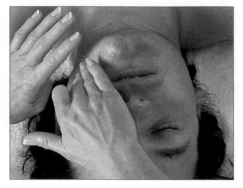

1 Make small, upwards circular movements all round the mouth with the tips of your middle fingers. Work with both hands simultaneously, and cross your thumbs to equalize the pressure of your hands.

2 Stroke with your fingertips from the upper lip, under the cheek-bones, to the ears. Then, still with your fingertips, stroke from the lower lip to the ears. These movements help to prevent lines round the mouth.

3 With your hands facing each other on one cheek, loosely roll your fingers up under the cheek-bone with one hand following the other. This releases tension in the jaw. Repeat on the other side.

MASSAGING THE FOREHEAD

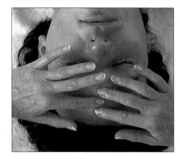 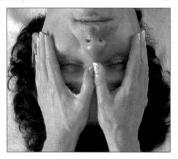 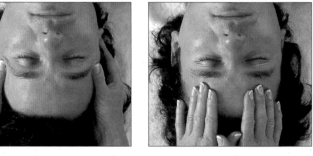

1 Put your hands across the forehead, and press firmly with the first two fingers of each hand. Make zig-zag strokes with your hands moving towards each other. Start with a small movement, then enlarge it to cover the whole forehead.

2 This soothing movement is very effective for reducing tension and relieving headaches. Place your thumbs on the bridge of the nose. Stroke out to the temples and press gently. Repeat the stroke a little higher up and gradually cover the whole forehead up to the hairline.

3 Make circular pressures all over the forehead with your fingers or thumbs. Work with both hands simultaneously from the centre to the temples, with smooth, rhythmic pressures. Upwards circles are energizing; downwards circles are soporific.

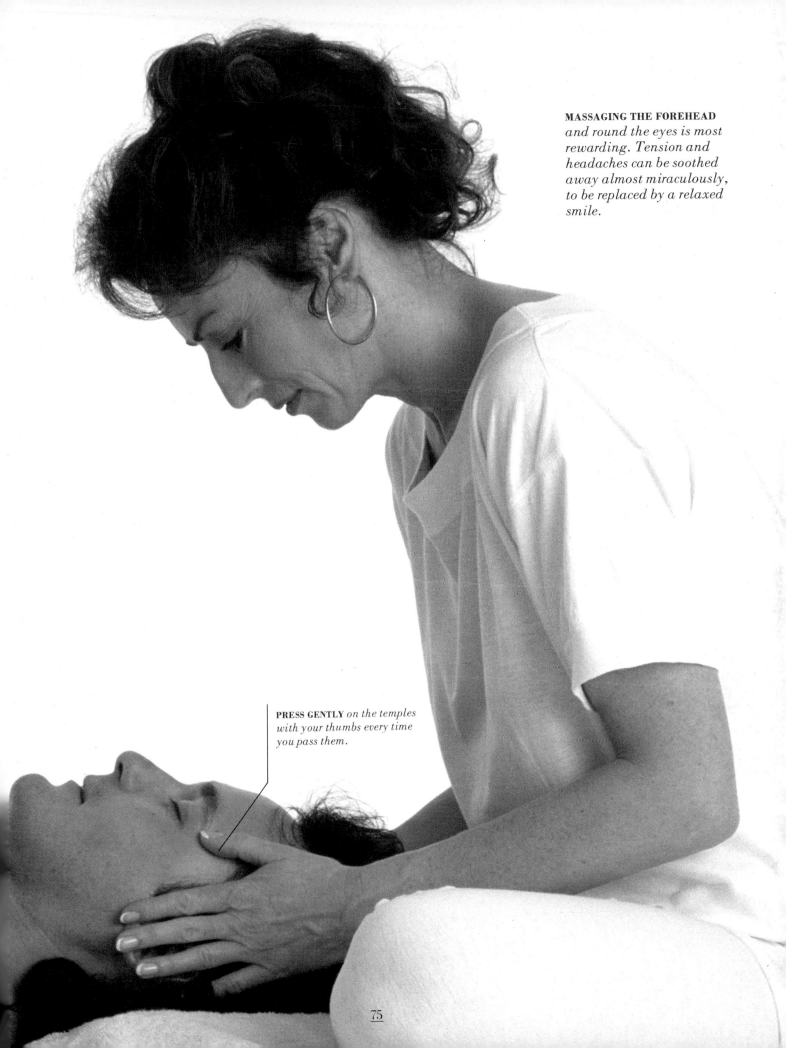

MASSAGING THE FOREHEAD *and round the eyes is most rewarding. Tension and headaches can be soothed away almost miraculously, to be replaced by a relaxed smile.*

PRESS GENTLY *on the temples with your thumbs every time you pass them.*

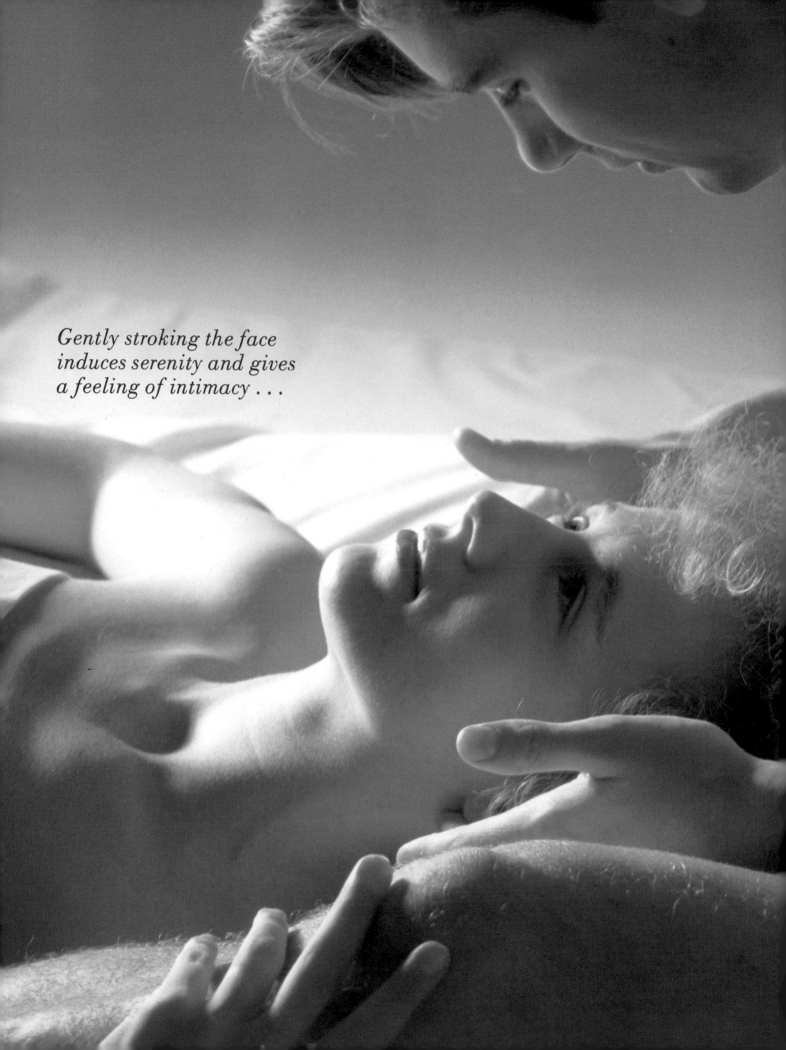

Gently stroking the face induces serenity and gives a feeling of intimacy . . .

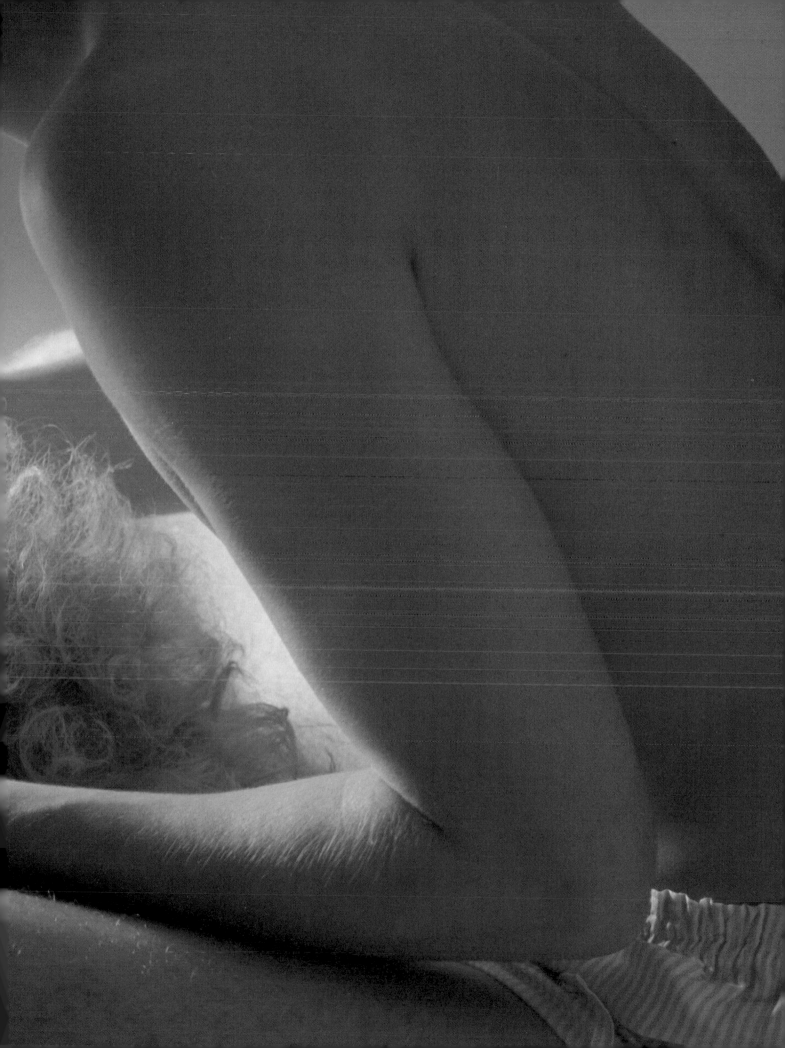

CIRCLING THE EYES
Starting at the bridge of the nose, stroke firmly out along the eyebrows with your fingertips. Circle on the temples then glide back very lightly under the eyes to the nose. Try this with your hands moving out simultaneously, then alternately. This is amazingly relaxing, obliterating all anxiety and tension.

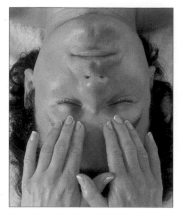

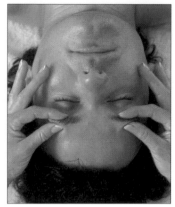

SQUEEZING THE EYEBROWS
This is a good contrast to the last stroking sequence. Squeeze the eyebrows between your thumbs and forefingers, starting at the bridge of the nose and working out to the temples. Press gently at the temples and then return your fingers through the air under the eyes and repeat.

EYE MASSAGE

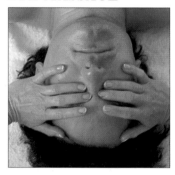

1 Place your fingers across the forehead, then slide them down until the middle and ring fingers rest lightly on the eyes. Pause for a moment, press very gently then separate the fingers and glide them out across the eyes. Press gently on the temples.

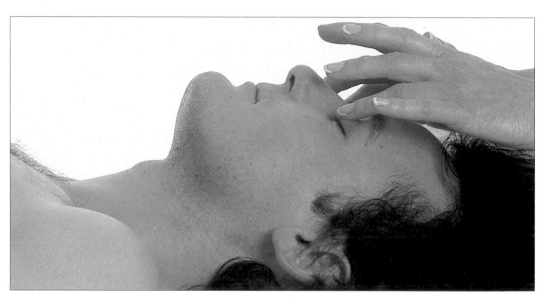

2 When you feel more confident about massaging the face, and your fingers are dexterous, you can try massaging the eyes lightly. Use your ring fingers to make circular pressures all over the eyelids. This can feel most relaxing, but with a heavy hand it can be rather uncomfortable.

ALTERNATE STROKING
This is my favourite of all the massage strokes. It is so comforting and, as is so often the case, the sheer simplicity of the movement makes it effective. Place one hand across the forehead and stroke up towards the hairline, moulding the hand around the forehead. Lift the hand away and begin stroking with the other hand, returning the first hand to start again.

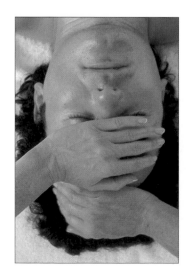

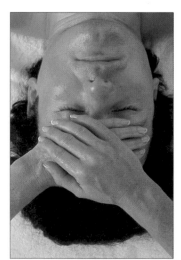

FINAL TOUCH
Cup your hands over the forehead. Hold them still for a couple of seconds, then slowly and gently press down. Hold the pressure for a moment then release it very, very gradually, so that your hands lift slowly away from the forehead. This simple technique seems to consolidate the whole face massage, and it feels as though you are pulling out the last vestiges of tension from the body.

HEAD MASSAGE

The perfect way of completing a face massage is to massage the head, spreading relaxation to every part of the body. There is a thin layer of muscle covering the skull, which tightens when we are tense, causing headaches and a feeling of anxiety. By relaxing this muscle, a head massage can be particularly effective at alleviating anxiety and relaxing the whole body.

When the scalp tightens, the blood supply to the hair follicles is restricted, and so they become undernourished. By stimulating the circulation,

massage can improve hair growth. It will not make a bald head suddenly sprout a thick growth, but it really can improve the condition of the hair. It is easy to massage your own head, and my clients who have massaged their scalps for ten minutes twice a day have noticed a definite improvement in the condition of their hair.

After you have finished massaging the face, remain kneeling behind the head, and flow smoothly into the head massage without adding any more oil.

ROTARY PRESSURES

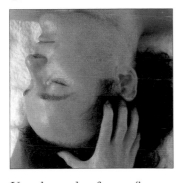

Use the pads of your fingers to make small circles all over the scalp. Start at the front and work over the whole head. Do extra work in the hollows at the base of the skull. Try to move the scalp around to release tension in the underlying muscles.

EAR MASSAGE

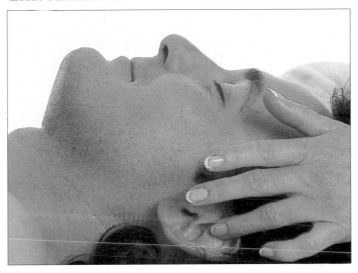

Squeeze the ears all over and make small circular pressures between your thumbs and forefingers. Then, with your ring fingers, slowly explore all the crevices and trace all round the ear.

NECK STRETCH

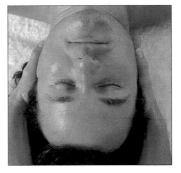

Place your hands behind the neck, with your little fingers on the skull and the others facing each other behind the neck. Gently and steadily pull the head towards you to stretch the neck. Keep the neck straight, and stretch it slowly and smoothly.

PULL THE HAIR

Start by simply stroking the hair, then grasp a bunch at the roots and pull it towards you. Though this may sound painful, it will not hurt at all if you grasp the hair right at the roots. Release your grasp and glide your fingers up the hair. Use your hands alternately as you pull and glide up the hair. This movement gives the lovely feeling of pulling away all tightness in the scalp.

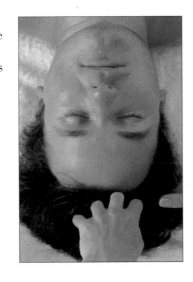

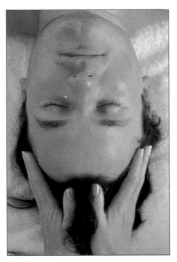

FINAL TOUCH

To finish the massage, place your hands on either side of the head, with your fingers covering the ears and the heels of your hands by the temples. Gently press your hands towards each other and hold for a couple of seconds. Release the pressure very slowly, then slide your hands up the sides of the head and glide them gently off the top. Repeat this movement a couple of times.

TEN-MINUTE MASSAGE

This quick, refreshing massage can be fitted in at any odd moment. It fits into anyone's schedule, however busy. Since it is not necessary to undress, you can do it at the office, while watching television, or even at a party. Your friend can sit astride a chair or on the floor, with you standing or kneeling behind.

1 Rest your forearms on the fleshy area on the top of the shoulders. Lean forwards so that your weight gently eases the shoulders down. This helps to break down some of the tension that makes the shoulders hunch up.

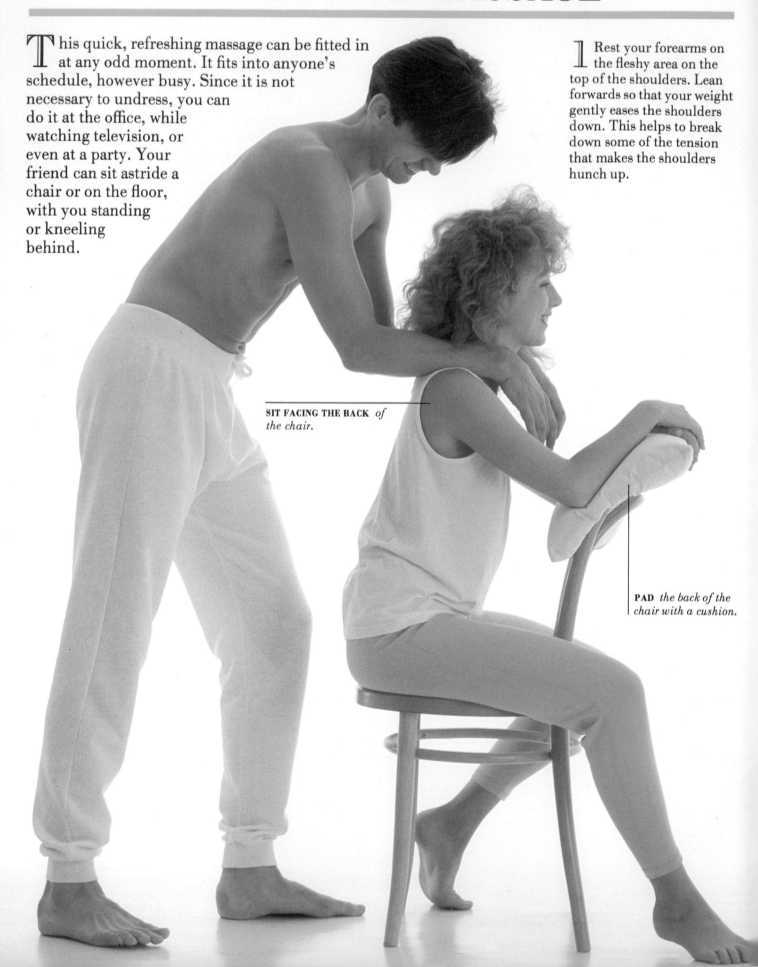

SIT FACING THE BACK *of the chair.*

PAD *the back of the chair with a cushion.*

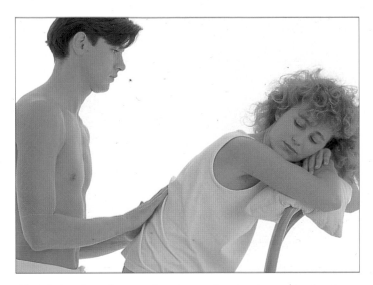

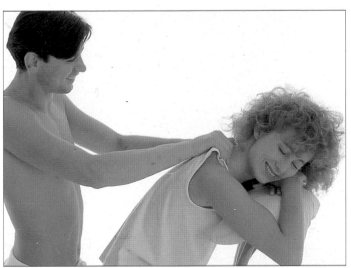

2 With relaxed, open hands stroke firmly up the back on either side of the spine. When you reach the shoulders, pull them down gently, then stroke out, curve your hands round the tops of the arms, and glide lightly down the sides. Repeat this about six times.

3 Knead the muscle across the top of the shoulders. Use both hands on one side, alternately squeezing and releasing the flesh. Work on both shoulders and out across the tops of the arms. It is a warming movement which helps to relax these taut muscles.

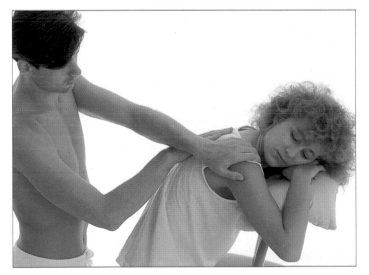

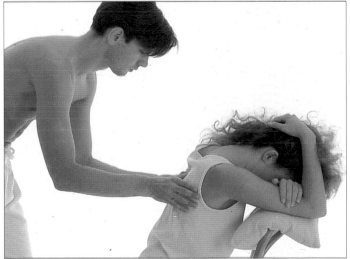

4 Now calm the area by stroking gently. Repeat the initial T-shaped stroke, then do extra work round the shoulders. Stroke in a circle over the top of one shoulder and round the top of the arm, with one hand following the other. Then work on the opposite shoulder.

5 Place your thumbs on either side of the spine and lean onto them. Hold the pressure for a few seconds, then glide up about an inch and repeat, working upwards from the lower back. When you reach the top, work out across the shoulders and round the shoulder blades.

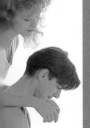
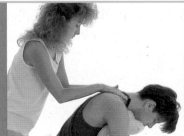
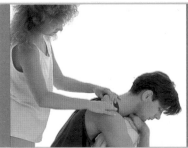
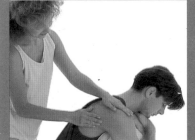
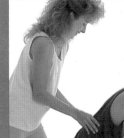

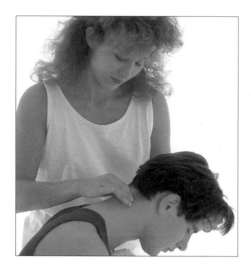

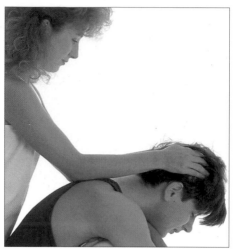

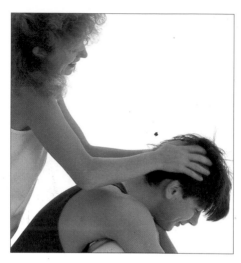

6 Support your friend's head with one hand and massage the back of his neck with the other. Stroke up the neck, then do circular pressures. Work thoroughly on the neck and round the base of the skull.

7 Now use both hands to make circular pressures all over the head. Do not pull the hair, but try to move the scalp around. Massage all over the head, around the ears, and on the temples and forehead.

8 Rub briskly back and forth all over the head with your finger-tips. This stimulating movement relieves tension, and leaves your friend alert and refreshed. Then glide your hands down to the shoulders.

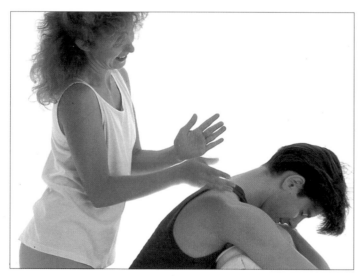

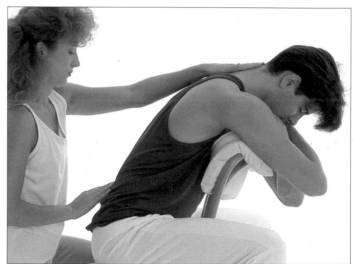

9 With open, very relaxed hands hack across the shoulders and upper back. This is an upwards springy movement, with your hands rhythmically bouncing up and down. The effect is lively and stimulating. Avoid the kidney area, and don't strike the spine itself.

10 Soothe the whole back by repeating the initial stroking, then flow into the cat stroke. Stroke down the back with one hand following the other in a lazy, monotonous rhythm. Finish with the feather stroke: use just your fingertips to stroke very lightly down the back.

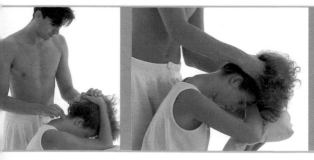

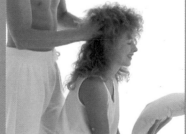

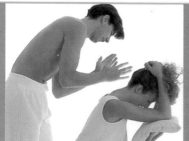

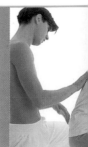

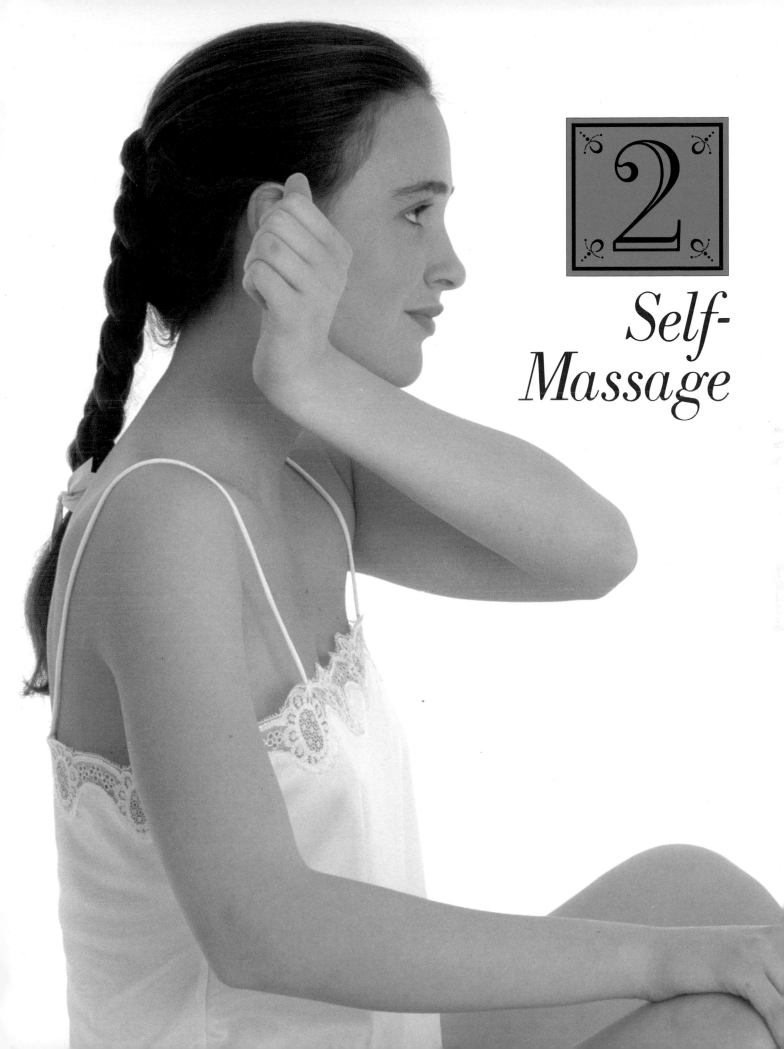

2

Self-Massage

ROUND THE BODY

If you cannot find anyone to give you a massage, you can easily massage yourself. This is not quite as enjoyable as being massaged by someone else, because you can never completely switch off, but if you work slowly and rhythmically, you will find that you can soothe away tension and practically send yourself to sleep. You alone know all your aches and pains, so you can use the healing power of self-massage to alleviate them.

You can massage yourself at any time and vary the massage to suit your needs by emphasizing either the fast, stimulating movements or the slow, soporific ones. Use self-massage to energize yourself before work in the morning, or to unwind in the evening. You can massage your feet while watching television, or massage your hands while talking to a friend. Even when driving, instead of fuming impatiently in a traffic jam, massage your neck and shoulders.

You do not need to undress, but you must be comfortable. Use oil if you are massaging on bare skin. Sit in a chair or on the floor, or lie down with your knees bent and your feet on the floor.

SHOULDERS

Most people suffer from occasional stiff necks, aching shoulders and head-aches, so the shoulders and neck are the perfect place to begin the self-massage. Also, since nearly everyone loves to have this area massaged, it is a good part of the body for trying out the various movements.

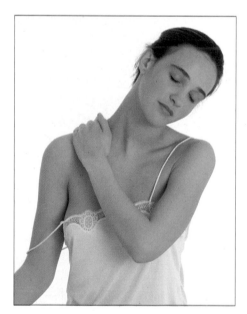

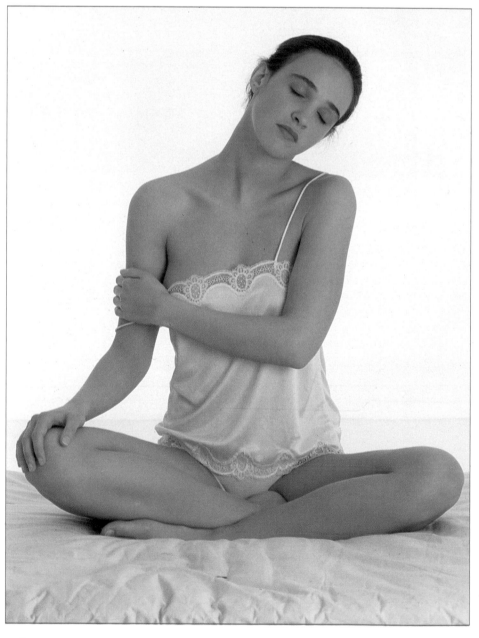

1 ▲▶ Stroke your right shoulder with your left hand. Mould your hand to the curves of your body: starting at the base of your skull, stroke down the side of your neck, over your shoulder and down your arm to the elbow. Glide back to your neck and repeat at least three times, then stroke the other side.

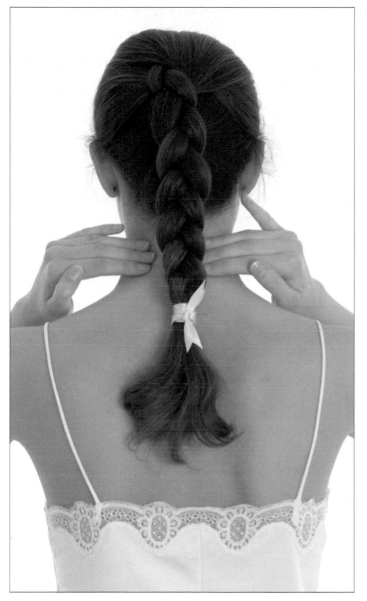

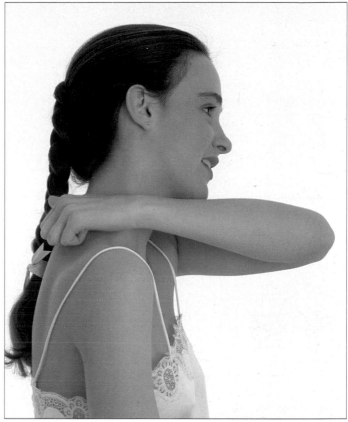

2 ◄Make circular pressures with your fingertips on either side of the spine. Work up the neck and around the base of the skull. Then knead each shoulder: squeeze and release the flesh on your shoulders and at the top of your arms.

3 ▲Loosely clench your left hand into a fist and rhythmically pound your right shoulder. Keep your wrist flexible. This lovely, springy movement improves the circulation and can be very invigorating if you are tired. Repeat on the other side.

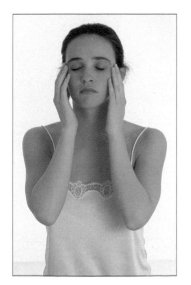

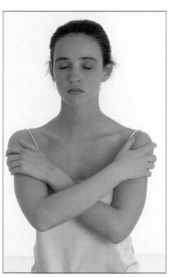

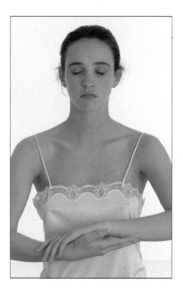

4 ◄◄◄Finish by stroking softly and smoothly with both hands. Start with your hands on the sides of your face, and glide them gently down under your chin. Slide your hands past each other at the front of the neck, so that each hand is on the opposite shoulder. Stroke gently over your shoulders, down your arms and off at your fingertips. Repeat as often as you like. This hypnotic stroke is incredibly relaxing and can relieve headaches.

LEGS

Knowing how to massage your own legs is very useful whether you lead an active or a sedentary life. Leg massage can relieve aching after standing for too long, and can help tired muscles recover after exercise. It stimulates the circulation and the lymphatic system (see page 141), and regular thigh massage can improve the appearance of the thighs by smoothing them out. Most of us have a little extra flesh on the thighs, and this makes massage easy. Do the whole sequence on one leg first, then work on the other one.

1 Start the massage by stroking your whole leg from ankle to thigh with one hand on each side of the leg. Begin at the foot and stroke smoothly up the calf, over the knee and up to the top of the thigh. Repeat about five times.

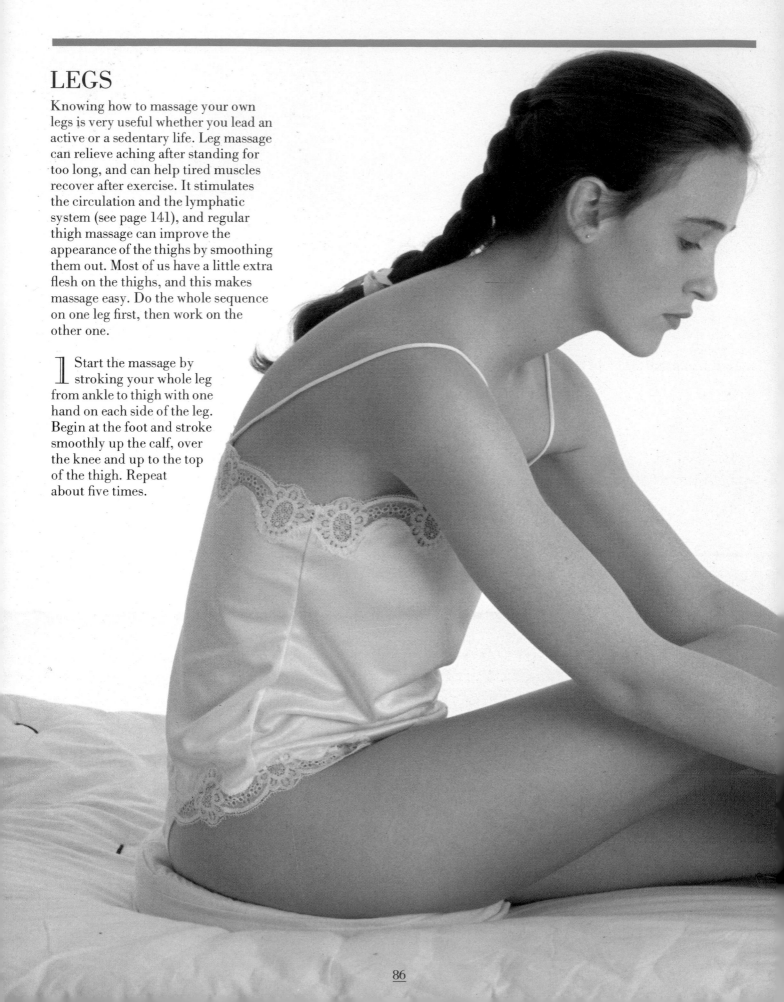

HANDS

It may seem surprising that people carry so much tension in their hands, but it's quite obvious when you think that we use our hands constantly. Most of our movements are holding, clutching actions, so it is very relaxing to counteract these by opening the palm and pulling the fingers.

1 ►Stroke the back of your hand, pushing firmly up towards the wrist, and gliding gently back. Then squeeze the hand all over, pressing it between your palm and your fingers.

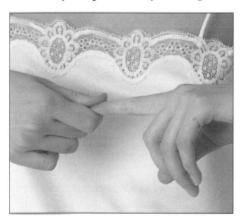

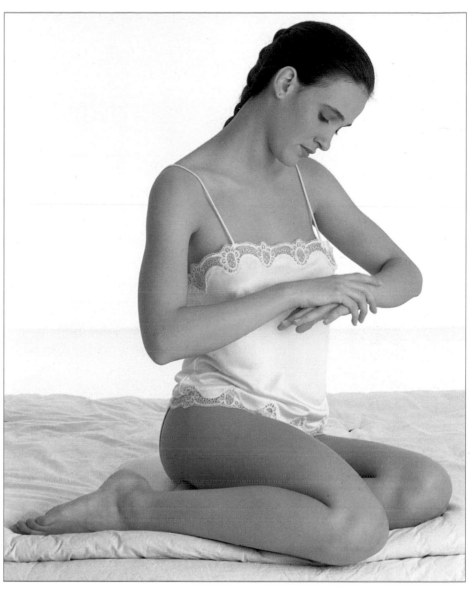

2 Squeeze each finger all over and make circular pressures over the joints with your thumb. Then hold the finger at its base and pull it gently to stretch it, sliding your grip up the finger and off the tip.

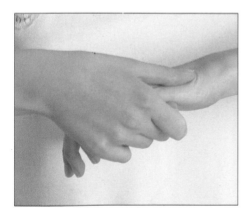

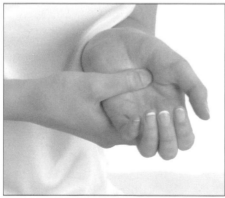

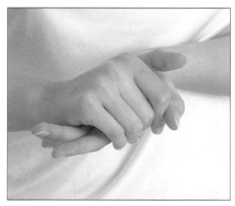

3 Stroke between the tendons on the back of the hand with your thumb. Start between the knuckles and stroke in the furrow to the wrist, doing four strokes in each furrow.

4 Turn your hand over and support the back with your fingers. Do firm circular and static pressures with your thumb, working all over the palm and round the wrist.

5 Finish the massage by stroking the palm of your hand from the fingers to the wrist. Push into it with the heel of your other hand, then glide gently back and repeat.

ARMS

Though you may feel tempted to ignore your arms, you will find that a thorough massage can help to release tension elsewhere in the body, especially in the shoulders.

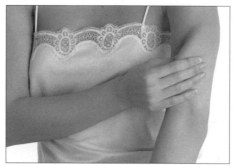

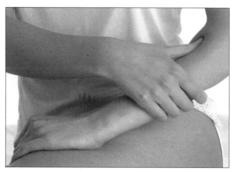

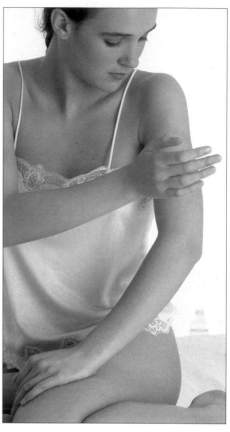

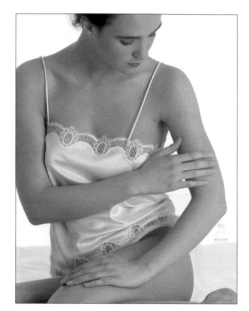

1 Soothe your whole arm by stroking from the wrist to the shoulder. Stroke firmly as you move up the arm, then glide back and repeat.

2 Knead all the way up your arm, squeezing and releasing the flesh. Pay particular attention to the fleshy area at the back of the upper arm.

3 Do circular pressures on your forearm with your thumb. Then, with your thumb and fingers, circle in all the hollows around the elbow.

4 Pat your upper arm to stimulate the circulation and help prevent the unhealthy look some arms have. Finally, stroke your whole arm again.

ABDOMEN

It is natural to rub your stomach when it aches, and any form of abdomen massage, however basic, is extremely comforting. Lie down to massage it, with your knees bent up.

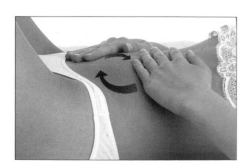

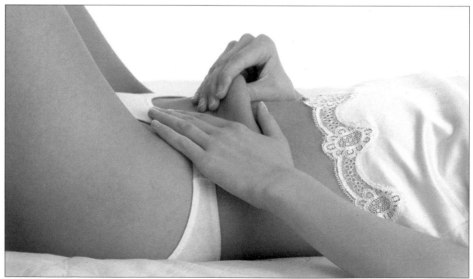

1 Stroke clockwise round your abdomen with one hand following the other in a circle, using the whole surface of your hands.

2 Knead all over your abdomen with your fingers and thumbs. Then roll onto your side to knead your hips and bottom. Turn onto your

back and stroke round your abdomen again. Cup your hands over your navel until you feel heat gathering, then lift them away slowly.

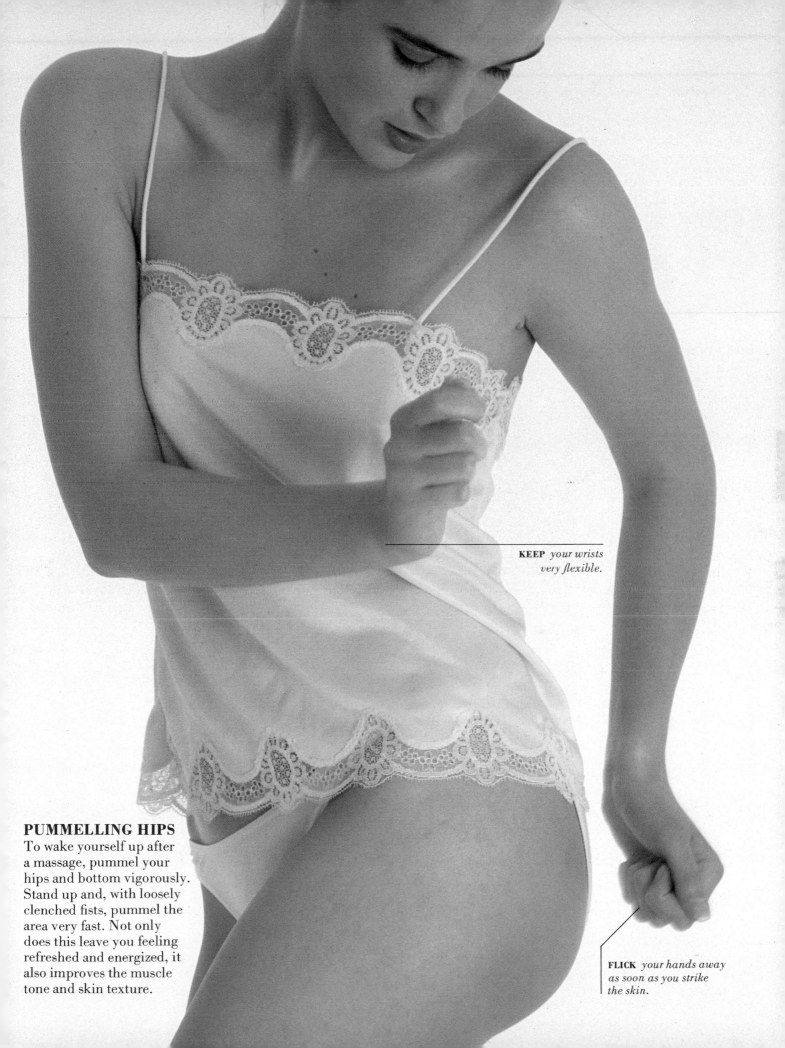

KEEP *your wrists very flexible.*

PUMMELLING HIPS
To wake yourself up after a massage, pummel your hips and bottom vigorously. Stand up and, with loosely clenched fists, pummel the area very fast. Not only does this leave you feeling refreshed and energized, it also improves the muscle tone and skin texture.

FLICK *your hands away as soon as you strike the skin.*

FACE AND NECK

Giving yourself a face massage can lift headaches, relieve anxiety and banish tiredness. Face massage can also benefit your appearance – improving your complexion and leaving your face looking fresher and younger. Use a fine face oil, so that you don't drag your skin. You can fit a massage in at any time: a stimulating one first thing in the morning, or a soothing one in the evening. Try varying the movements: brisk and fast for an energizing effect, or slow and smooth if you want to calm yourself down. Repeat each movement as often as you like.

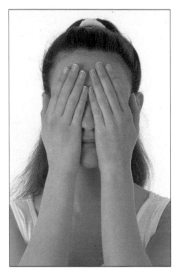 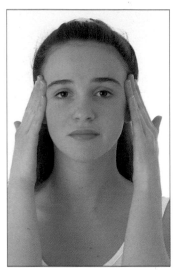

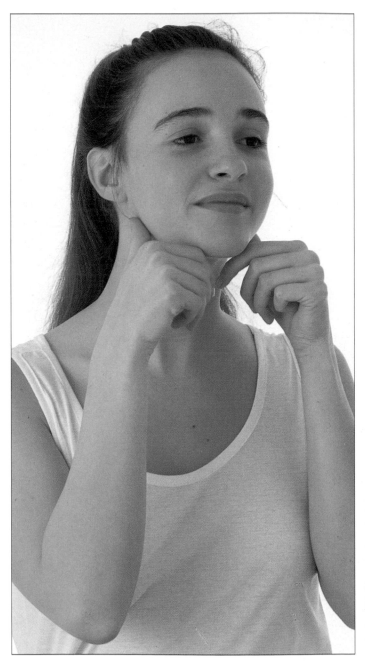

1 Start by putting your hands over your face, with your fingers on your forehead and the heels of your hands on your chin. Hold them there for a moment, then very slowly and gently draw them out towards your ears. As they move out, imagine that they are dissolving all the tension from your face and drawing it away like magnets.

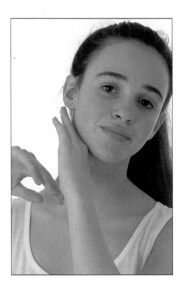 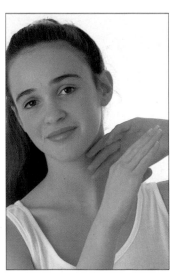

2 Tilt your head to one side and, using the back of your hands, stroke from the collar-bone to the chin, one hand following the other. Tilt your head to the left and stroke up the right side of your neck, then repeat on the other side. Stroke firmly to stimulate the circulation and help keep your neck looking young.

3 Pinch all along your jawline using your thumbs and the knuckles of your index fingers. Start under your chin and work out to your ears. Keep the pinching close to the bone, so that you don't stretch the skin. One of my clients, who is a great beauty, swears that this movement has prevented her developing a double chin.

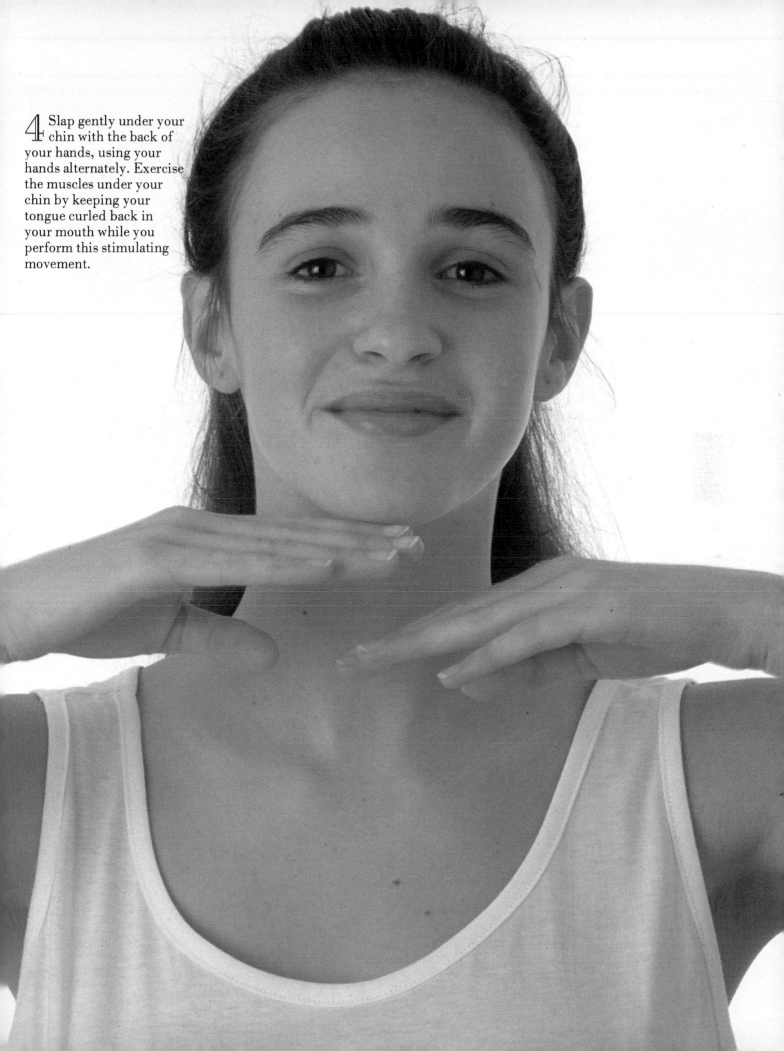

4 Slap gently under your chin with the back of your hands, using your hands alternately. Exercise the muscles under your chin by keeping your tongue curled back in your mouth while you perform this stimulating movement.

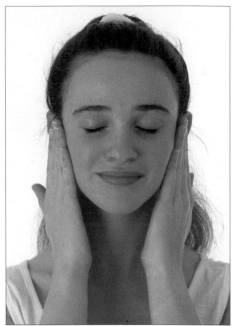

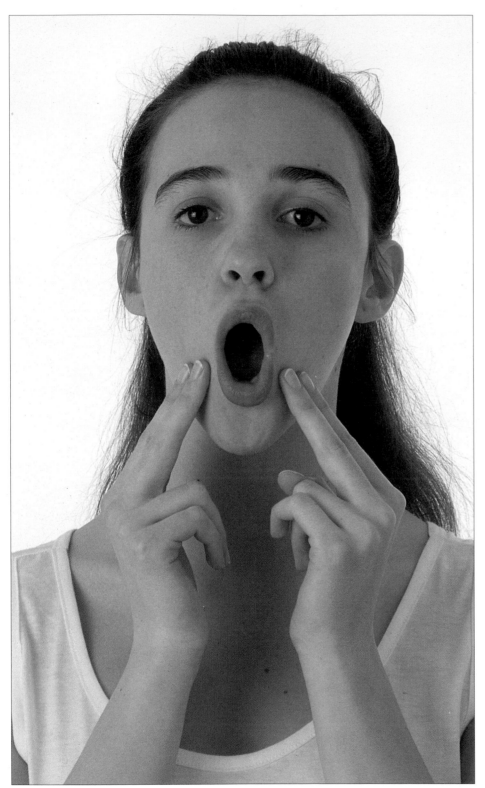

6 Stroke from the corners of your mouth to your ears. Use one hand on each cheek and move them both out together. Then, both hands on one side, stroke from your mouth to your ear, using the back of your fingers.

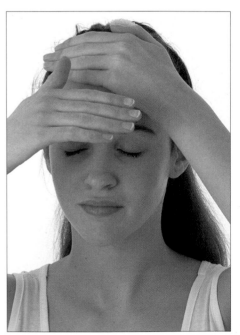

5 Make small circular pressures all over your chin and round your mouth with the index and middle fingers of each hand. While you do this, exercise the muscle round your mouth by making a large 'O' and holding your lips tightly over your teeth. Then exercise the muscle further by exaggeratedly saying 'aah, ooh, eee, uu' to stimulate the circulation and help to prevent little wrinkles developing round your mouth.

7 Stroke up your forehead from the bridge of your nose to your hairline, with one hand following the other. Mould your hands to the shape of your forehead, and close your eyes to enjoy this soothing movement.

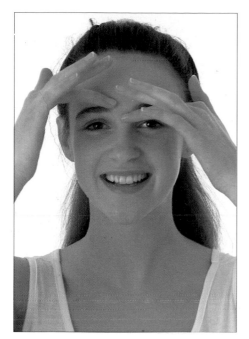

8 Massage the muscle between your eyebrows to counteract frown lines. Put both index fingers on the bridge of your nose and make short, firm strokes, upwards first, then across, and then diagonally.

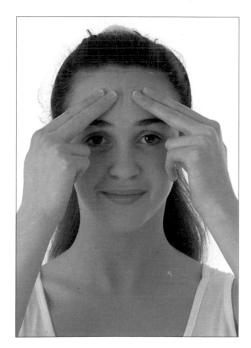

9 Make circular pressures all over your forehead, working in lines from the bridge of your nose to your temples, to cover the whole forehead up to your hairline. Press firmly, but do not drag your skin.

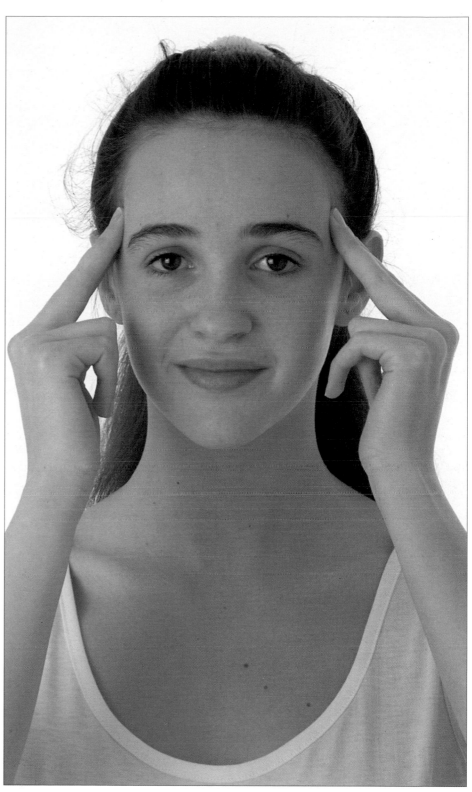

10 Stroke your forehead gently with your fingertips to soothe it after the last stimulating movement. Stroke from the centre of your forehead to your temples, and finish by pressing gently on the temples.

You can strengthen your jaw muscle by clenching your teeth slightly as you press on the temples. Feel the muscle working under your fingers. Then, hardly moving the skin, circle slowly and steadily to stimulate the muscle.

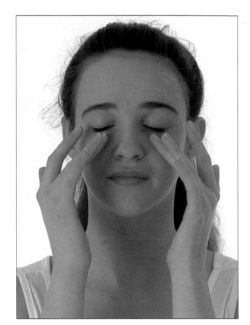

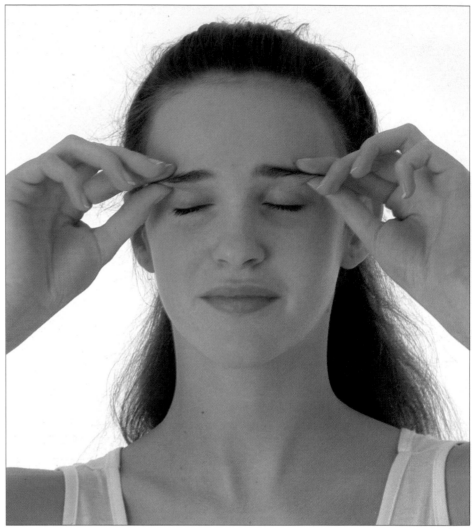

11 Stroke in a circle round your eyes with your middle fingers. Stroke firmly from the bridge of your nose out over your eyebrows, press on your temples, then glide lightly under your eyes, barely touching the skin.

12 ▶Pinch along your eyebrows from the centre to the temples with your thumbs and index fingers. Then press into the tiny indentation in the bone under the eyebrows at the bridge of the nose.

13 ▶Relax your eyes by palming. Put the heel of your hands into your eye sockets, and hold your hands there for a few seconds, enjoying the blackness. Press gently, then slowly glide your hands away.
   Many actors and actresses tell me that when they are utterly exhausted, but still have to go on stage for the final act, they palm their eyes like this. After only a few seconds of blackness, there is a wonderful light which revitalizes them. Do try this: it only takes a few seconds, but it is remarkably refreshing.

14 ▶▶Finish by covering your face with your hands and stroking gently out to the sides. This simple massage should make your skin look fresher and you will feel revitalized.

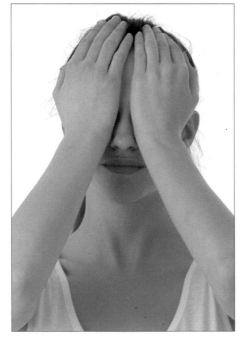

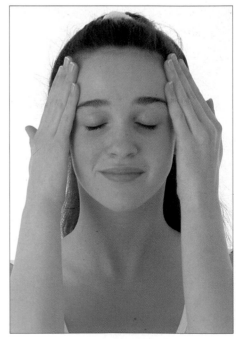

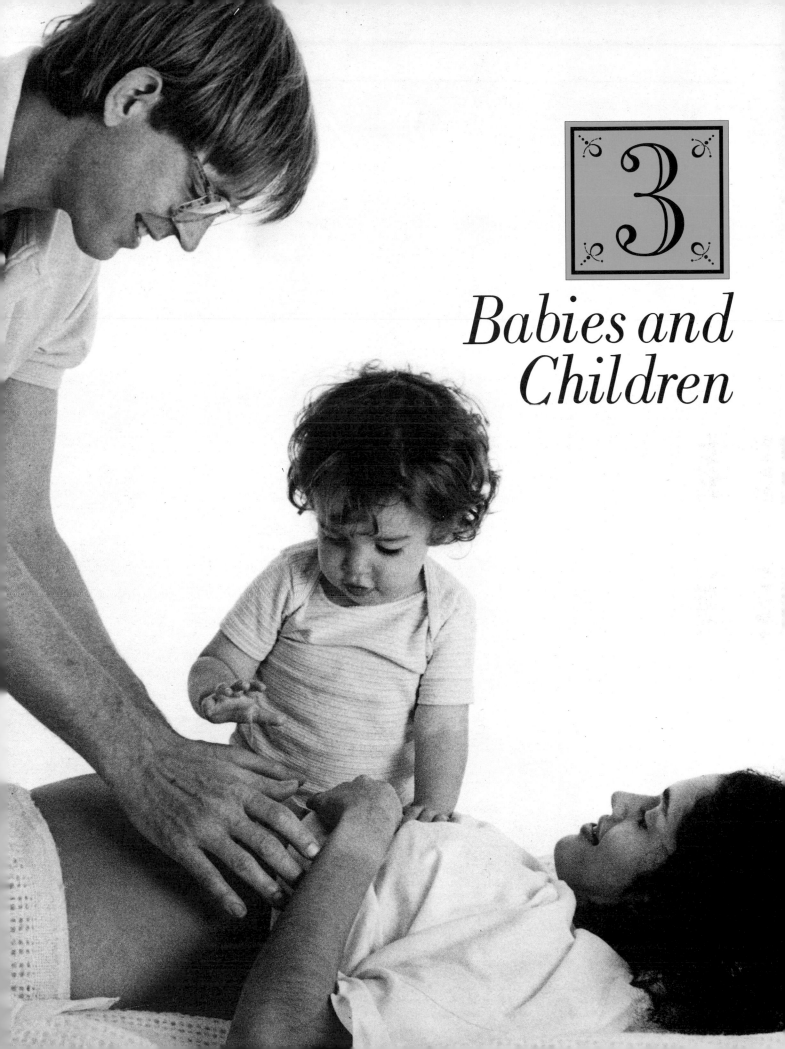

3

Babies and Children

HAVING A BABY

I massage my clients throughout pregnancy, and think that careful, gentle massage would benefit all pregnant women. However, if you are pregnant and would like to be massaged, or if you want to massage someone who is pregnant, I would advise you to check with a doctor before you start.

As well as being extremely relaxing, massage can alleviate many of the minor complaints, such as backache and insomnia, which are common during pregnancy. Clients frequently tell me that the only time they sleep properly is after a massage, when they are completely relaxed.

When massaging a pregnant woman, all your movements should be very smooth and gentle, and you should avoid deep pressures and percussion techniques altogether. You can massage softly on the abdomen itself, and even the unborn baby seems to appreciate this. One friend said that the only time her stomach did not feel like a football pitch was after a massage. She was sure that the baby was lulled to sleep by it.

In many parts of the world, massage is used at all stages of pregnancy, and even before conception to increase the fertility of women. In Nigeria, for instance, women who have been unable to

ABDOMEN MASSAGE

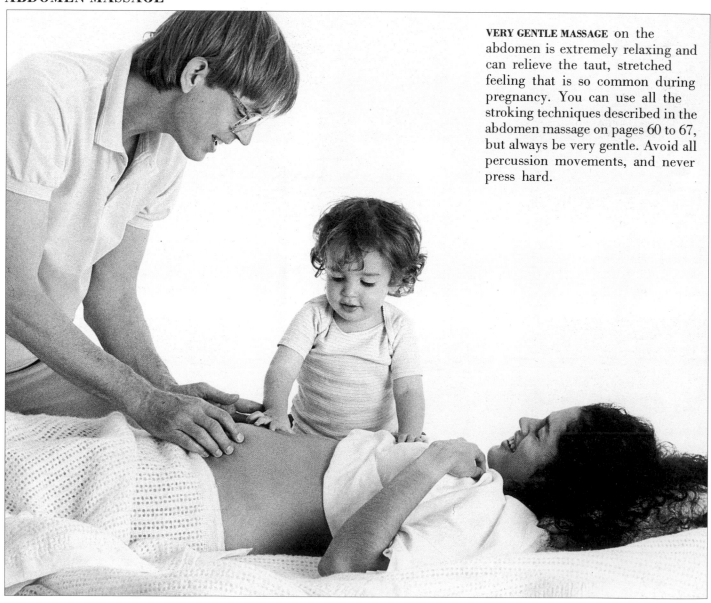

VERY GENTLE MASSAGE on the abdomen is extremely relaxing and can relieve the taut, stretched feeling that is so common during pregnancy. You can use all the stroking techniques described in the abdomen massage on pages 60 to 67, but always be very gentle. Avoid all percussion movements, and never press hard.

conceive visit a specially trained masseuse who massages the lower abdomen. One girl who had been barren for years told me that she was able to conceive after three weeks of daily massage. The masseuses are usually the local midwives, and in Africa, India and Malaysia I have frequently been told that they are able to change the position of the baby to make the birth easier.

GIVING A MASSAGE

Give a complete body massage (see Chapter 1, pages 22 to 79), spending extra time on the legs, back and abdomen, which are the areas that most

commonly feel uncomfortable during pregnancy. Concentrate on any areas where you feel tension – usually the lower back or shoulders. If the doctor advises you not to massage these areas, you can still help your partner to relax by massaging her face, arms, hands and feet.

Use plenty of cushions to make your partner comfortable. When she is lying on her back, put cushions under her knees to relax her abdomen and reduce the curve in her lower back. She may also like to have cushions under her head and shoulders. For the back massage, she can lie on her side or sit astride a chair.

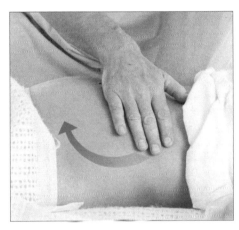

1 Kneel beside your partner and stroke clockwise round her abdomen with one hand, keeping the stroke smooth and gentle.

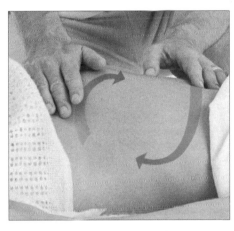

2 Continue stroking clockwise round the abdomen, but now use both hands, one following the other smoothly in a gentle, flowing stroke.

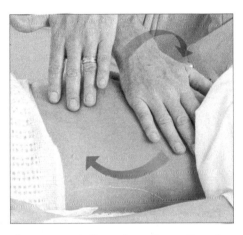

3 Make a full circle with one hand and a half circle with the other, lifting one hand over your other arm as your arms cross.

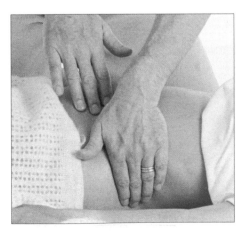

4 Stroke gently up the side of the waist, one hand after the other. Lift your hands off as they reach the navel and start again.

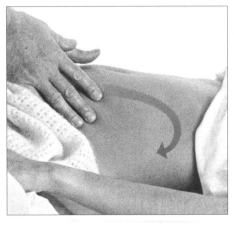

5 Stroke up the abdomen very gently and glide down the sides. Gradually stroke more softly, until you are barely touching the skin.

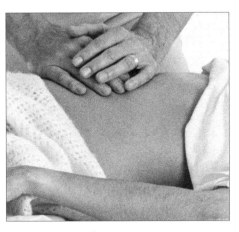

6 Cup your hands over the navel for a few seconds until you feel heat gathering underneath, then lift your hands very slowly away.

LEG MASSAGE

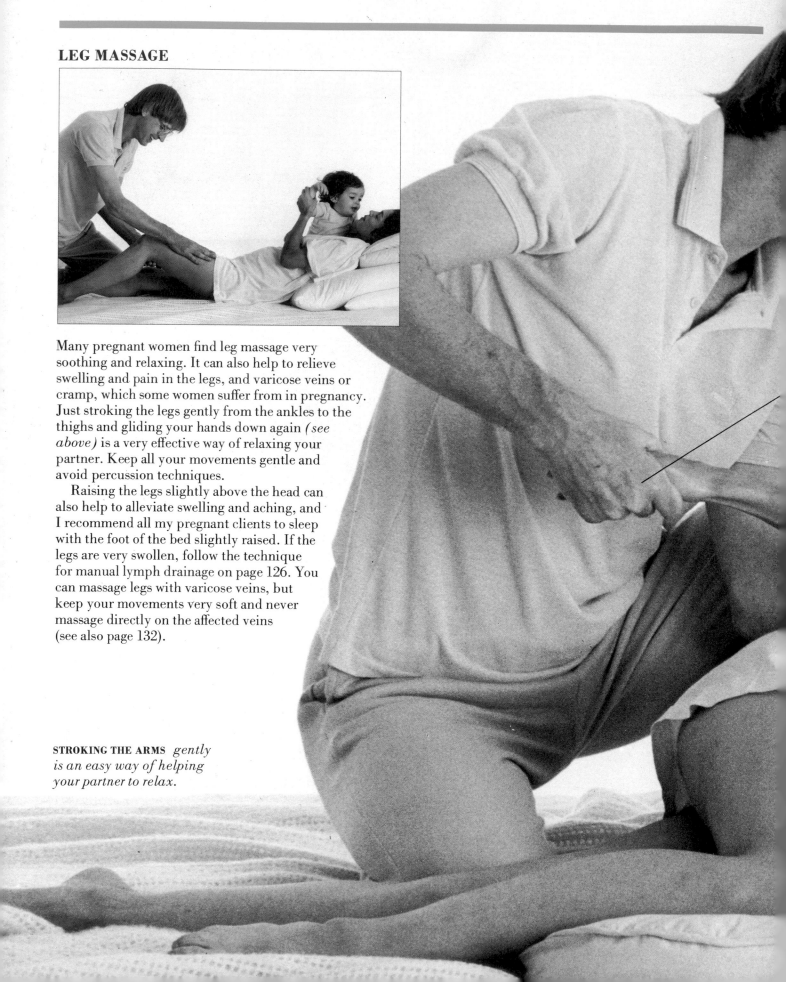

Many pregnant women find leg massage very
soothing and relaxing. It can also help to relieve
swelling and pain in the legs, and varicose veins or
cramp, which some women suffer from in pregnancy.
Just stroking the legs gently from the ankles to the
thighs and gliding your hands down again *(see
above)* is a very effective way of relaxing your
partner. Keep all your movements gentle and
avoid percussion techniques.

Raising the legs slightly above the head can
also help to alleviate swelling and aching, and
I recommend all my pregnant clients to sleep
with the foot of the bed slightly raised. If the
legs are very swollen, follow the technique
for manual lymph drainage on page 126. You
can massage legs with varicose veins, but
keep your movements very soft and never
massage directly on the affected veins
(see also page 132).

STROKING THE ARMS *gently
is an easy way of helping
your partner to relax.*

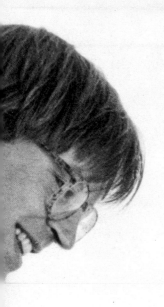

ARM MASSAGE▼

A very gentle arm massage is extremely soothing, and if you are advised against massaging her abdomen, this is an effective way of relaxing your partner. Some pregnant women feel dizzy if they lie on their backs for a long time. If your partner is affected in this way, she can lie on her side while you massage her arms. You can follow the complete sequence for massaging the arms (see pages 54 to 59), or simply stroke her arms slowly and rhythmically.

BACK MASSAGE

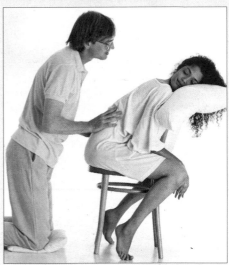

Backache is probably the most common complaint during pregnancy, and a back massage can relieve much of this discomfort. Your partner can either lie on her side or sit astride a chair, leaning on a cushion (see above). Follow the sequence given on pages 22 to 36, but do not apply deep pressures to the lower back during the first three months of pregnancy. Use plenty of stroking movements because they are very calming. Even morning sickness can sometimes be alleviated with massage: work firmly on the mid back from just above the waist to between the shoulder blades.

HOLD HER HAND *to support her arm.*

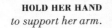

MOULD YOUR HAND *round her arm as you stroke.*

PUT CUSHIONS *under her head to help her neck and shoulders to relax.*

PUT A CUSHION *under the knee of her upper leg to make her more comfortable.*

DURING CHILDBIRTH

Being calming and reassuring, massage can be of immense value during childbirth. It can diminish backache, and is a positive way of comforting and supporting your partner. You can help her relax by massaging her back, shoulders, neck and feet, but don't massage her abdomen. When you massage her back and shoulders, your partner can lie on her side or sit astride a chair. Practise these movements beforehand so that you will be familiar with them.

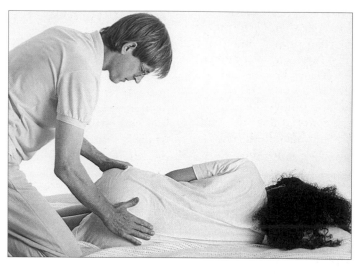

BACK MASSAGE

1 ▶Stroke all round the sacrum at the base of the spine with the heel of one hand, then stroke the lower back. Keep the movement smooth and flowing.

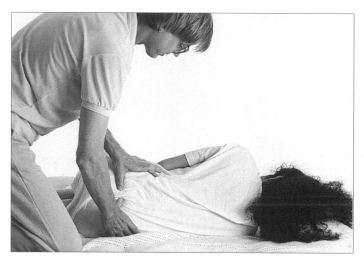

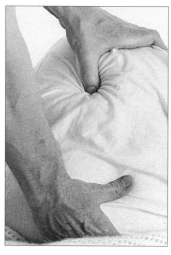

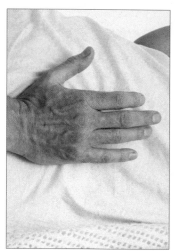

2 Do penetrating circular pressures with your thumbs all over the sacrum. Press firmly on this bony area and circle the skin over the underlying bone. Rest your fingers on your partner's hips to support them as you press.

3 Press deeply with your thumbs into the centre of each buttock. This can relieve lower back pain.

4 Apply a deep, firm pressure on the sacrum with the heel of one hand, to ease lower back pain.

FACE MASSAGE

During a lull between contractions, a gentle massage on the face is calming and reassuring. You can use any of the techniques shown on pages 72 to 78; the most relaxing are those round the eyes and on the forehead. Stroking up the forehead into the hairline is one of the best ways of reducing tension. Stroke gently, one hand following the other in a smooth, rhythmic sequence.

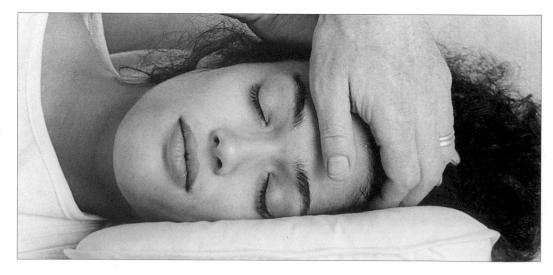

FOOT MASSAGE

Firm, deep massage on the feet can be of great benefit. The two techniques given below are the most useful during labour, and can help to relieve the pain of the contractions, although you can also do the complete sequence shown on pages 38 to 41.

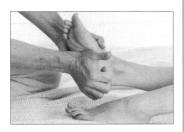

1 Support the foot with one hand and stroke the sole firmly with the heel of your other hand.

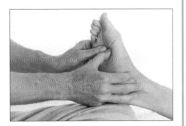

2 Apply deep pressures with your thumbs in a line down the centre of the sole to the heel.

SHIATSU POINTS

These points can relieve pain during childbirth and speed up delivery.

■ On the outside of the little toe, at the base of the nail (Bladder 67).

■ In the groove behind the shin bone, four finger widths above the ankle prominence on the inside of the leg (Spleen 6).

AFTER CHILDBIRTH

Massage is tremendously beneficial after childbirth. In parts of the East it is the tradition for a new mother to be cosseted and pampered, and every day for 40 days the local midwife massages her whole body, giving a particularly deep massage to the abdomen. A mother in Borneo told me how comforting she found this. "It felt as though my whole insides were being pushed back into place." After a month her stomach was flat, she had no aches and she felt energetic and lively.

How civilized these traditions seem compared with our own way of life. Every new mother would benefit from a regular massage. It eases the strain of caring for the baby, relieves the aches from picking up and carrying, reduces nervousness and stress and, above all, ensures at least an hour of complete relaxation. This would benefit the rest of the family too, because after the massage the mother would be filled with a sense of well-being. In fact one of the reasons that I first became interested in massage was because my mother was always in such a wonderful mood after having a massage. To give a massage, follow the sequence in Chapter 1, paying extra attention to the abdomen.

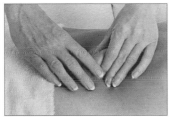

2 Knead firmly on the hips, then work gently across the abdomen in rows to cover the whole area.

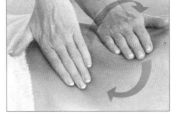

3 Stroke clockwise in a large circle round the abdomen, one hand following the other.

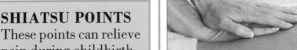

5 Stroke slowly up the abdomen with one hand on top of the other, starting at the pubic bone. Press firmly with the heel of your hands, reduce the pressure when you reach the navel and glide back down. Repeat several times.

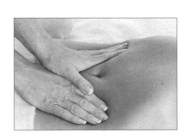

6 Put your hands together on the lower abdomen, with each thumb overlapping the other hand to make a large V. Scoop up with the outside edges of your hands, and stroke slowly and firmly from the pubic bone to the navel.

ABDOMEN MASSAGE

Ask your partner's doctor how soon you can start massaging her abdomen. The area may be rather tender, so massage with great care. Ask your partner to guide you, and avoid any movements that are painful. Don't massage the scar area after a Caesarean.

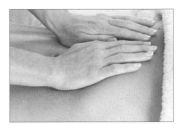

1 Stroke up the abdomen, then glide your hands down the sides. Repeat at least six times.

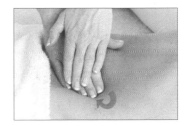

4 Do gentle circular pressures clockwise round the abdomen, one hand on top of the other.

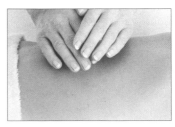

7 Finish the massage by stroking the abdomen very softly and gently, then cup your hands over the navel and hold them there for a few seconds until you feel heat gathering underneath. Then lift them away very, very slowly.

BABY MASSAGE

It is a natural reaction for parents to stroke, cuddle and caress their babies, and there is increasing evidence to show that massage is beneficial to a baby's health and well-being. The eminent obstetrician, Mr Yehudi Gordon, says: "Massage helps to reduce colic, constipation or diarrhoea, coughs, colds and irritability. It is a very powerful means of communicating in a non-verbal way, thus creating a strong link between mother, father and the baby." It is this strong link, or bonding, that many mothers remark on when they massage their babies. A daily massage allows time for the parent and the baby to become intimately acquainted.

Difficult babies can be quietened and lulled to sleep with a massage. One friend had a baby who suffered from convulsions, and she found that by massaging the baby's stomach each night she was able to calm her. Her daughter is now nine years old and healthy, but my friend still uses massage to soothe her if she gets agitated.

Babies have such wonderfully silky skin that they are a joy to touch, and indeed massage is as beneficial for the person giving the massage as it is for the baby. One client, who had severe "post-natal blues", found that massaging her baby was the only thing that cheered her up and helped her cope with caring for the baby.

GIVING A MASSAGE

There are no special techniques and no definite sequence for massaging babies, it is just a question of adapting a massage to fit their tiny bodies. As the body is so small, you will probably use the stroking movements most often. Stroke with your fingertips or your thumbs if the area you are working on is too small for the whole surface of your hands. You don't need to adhere strictly to the sequence below: you will quickly find out what your baby enjoys. Keep all your movements slow and smooth; let your hands be your guide and do whatever comes naturally.

Use a light vegetable oil for the whole massage, including the face. Almond oil or sunflower oil is easily available and suitable for babies. Baby oil is a mineral oil, and therefore is not easily absorbed by the skin.

FACE MASSAGE

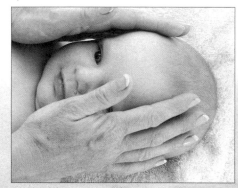 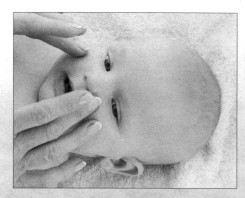

1 Stroke your baby's forehead from the centre to the sides. Then stroke from his nose out to the temples and glide down the sides to his chin.

2 Circle round his eyes, stroking out along the eyebrows and very gently back under the eyes. Then press very softly on the temples.

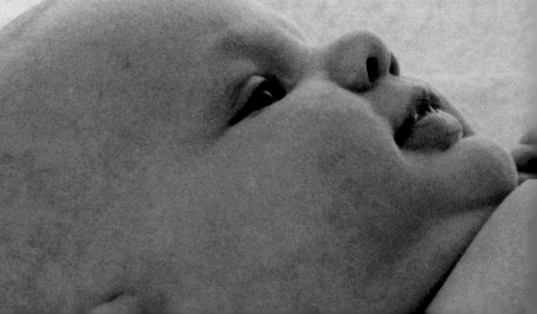

ABDOMEN MASSAGE

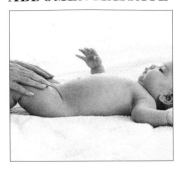
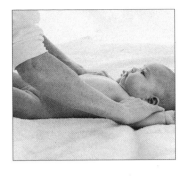
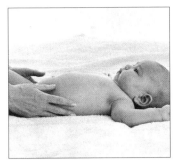

1 ◀◀◀Stroke from the thighs up the front of the body, glide your hands out to the shoulders, down the arms then down the sides of the body. Work with both hands together, then alternately – one hand stroking up as the other glides down.

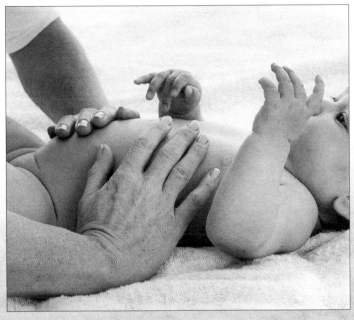

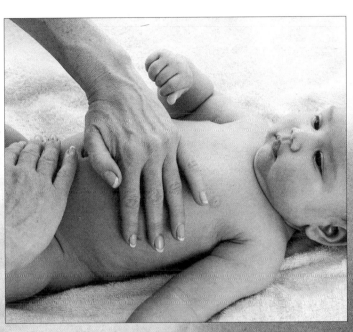

2 Put one hand on either side of the abdomen with your fingers pointing towards each other. Glide your hands back and forth across the abdomen in a criss-crossing movement, keeping the stroke across the abdomen light.

3 Stroke clockwise in a circle round the navel with one hand following the other. Lift one hand over your other arm as your arms cross. This soothing movement can relieve colic and stomach aches.

YOUR BABY *should be relaxed and comfortable, not hungry or too tired. After a bath is an ideal time. He can lie on your lap or on a towel on the floor. Make sure that the room is very warm and free from draughts.*

ARMS AND LEGS

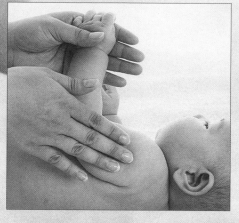

1 Hold up one arm and stroke down from the shoulder to the hand, then squeeze it gently all over.

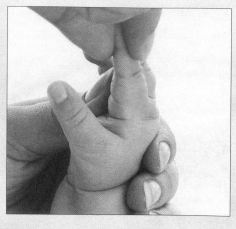

2 Stroke the back of your baby's hand, then uncurl the fingers and gently squeeze and rotate each finger.

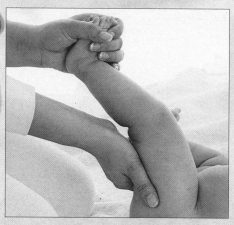

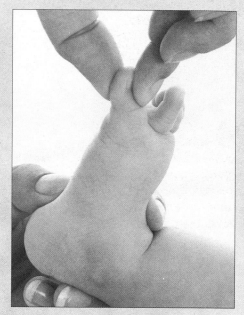

3 Lift one leg up and stroke and squeeze it all over.

4 ▶Stroke the foot, then squeeze and rotate each toe.

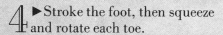

BABIES ARE FASCINATED *by their hands and feet, and will love to watch as you gently squeeze their fingers.*

BACK MASSAGE

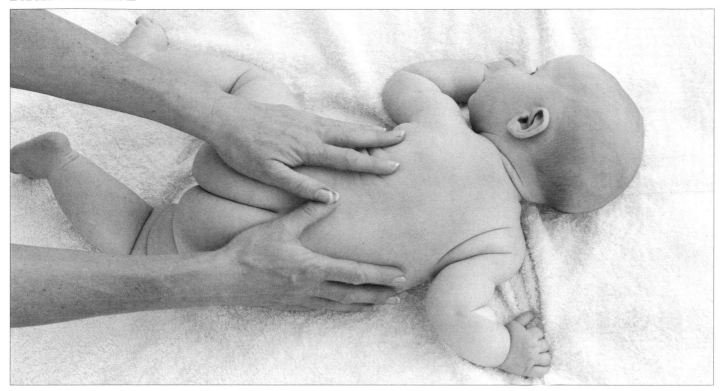

1 ▲ Turn your baby over onto his front and stroke the whole back. Start at the feet, stroke up the back of the legs, over the bottom and up the back. Glide your hands out across the shoulders and down the arms, then slide them gently down the sides.

2 ▶ Stroke with your thumbs up the back on either side of the spine.

3 ▶▶ Glide your hands gently back and forth across the back in a criss-crossing movement.

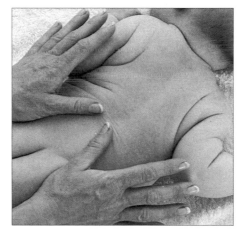

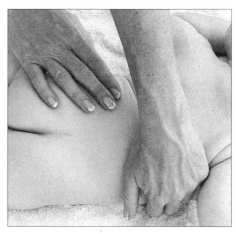

4 ▶ Stroke round each buttock and knead it gently, then rhythmically pat and pinch your baby's bottom softly, using your hands alternately. Surprisingly, most babies love this gentle patting, and as the skin is so satiny smooth, it is lovely to touch.

5 ▶▶ Finish the back massage with the cat stroke. Glide your hands very softly and smoothly down the back, one hand following the other. As one hand reaches the legs, lift it off, return it to the neck and repeat.

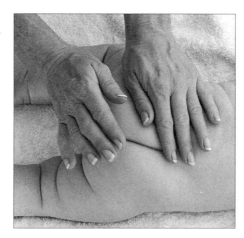

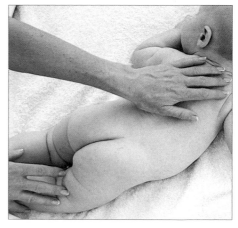

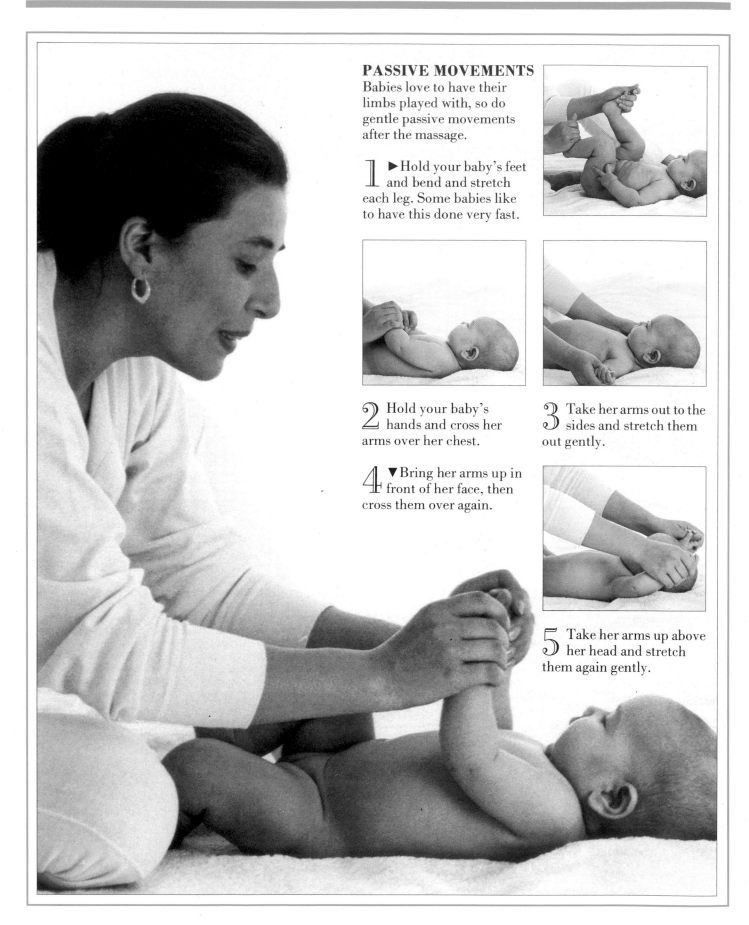

PASSIVE MOVEMENTS

Babies love to have their limbs played with, so do gentle passive movements after the massage.

1 ▶Hold your baby's feet and bend and stretch each leg. Some babies like to have this done very fast.

2 Hold your baby's hands and cross her arms over her chest.

3 Take her arms out to the sides and stretch them out gently.

4 ▼Bring her arms up in front of her face, then cross them over again.

5 Take her arms up above her head and stretch them again gently.

MASSAGE FOR CHILDREN

Massaging children is just as easy as massaging babies. Children of all ages thoroughly enjoy massage. They appreciate attention from adults and respond well to the relaxing strokes. There are no rules to follow when massaging a child – it depends on what your child enjoys. Experiment with some of the suggestions given here to find out what your child likes best. Some children become restless quite quickly, so just give a shorter treatment. As long as it is spontaneous and enjoyable, massage will benefit both you and your child. It can be part of a game or a restful part of a rough and tumble session. Your child need not undress – you can massage through light clothes.

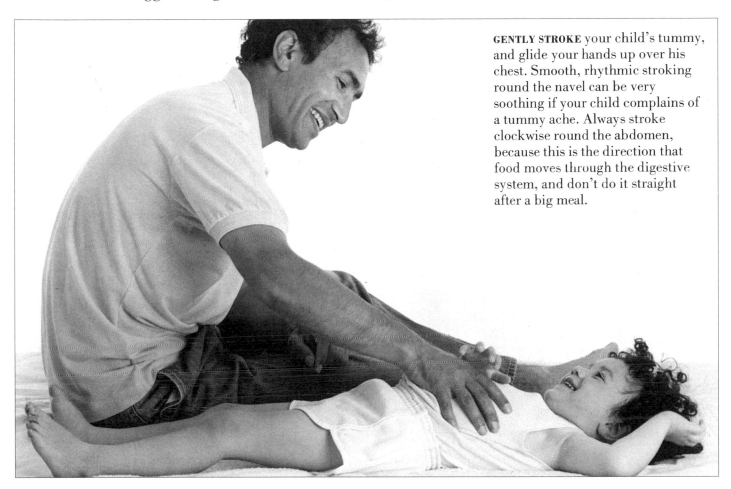

GENTLY STROKE your child's tummy, and glide your hands up over his chest. Smooth, rhythmic stroking round the navel can be very soothing if your child complains of a tummy ache. Always stroke clockwise round the abdomen, because this is the direction that food moves through the digestive system, and don't do it straight after a big meal.

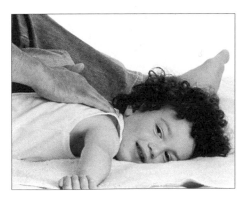

Stroke up your child's back and glide down the sides. Gently knead his shoulders, then stroke out over the tops of his arms.

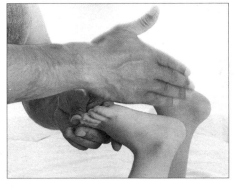

Stroke and squeeze down his legs, then massage his feet. Try hacking the soles: hold one foot up with one hand, and hack lightly with the other hand.

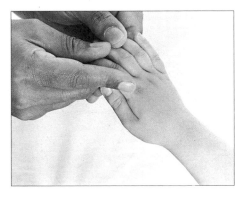

To massage his hands, squeeze and rotate each finger in turn, then stroke his palm. With little ones, you can make this into a counting game.

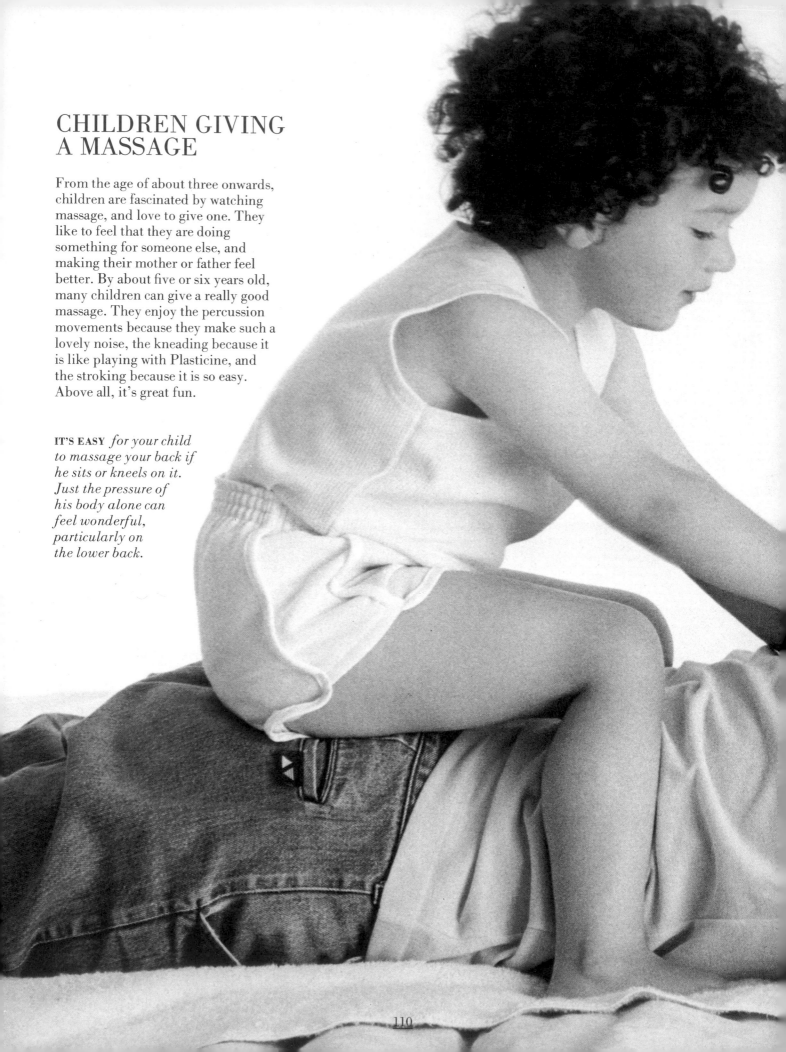

CHILDREN GIVING A MASSAGE

From the age of about three onwards, children are fascinated by watching massage, and love to give one. They like to feel that they are doing something for someone else, and making their mother or father feel better. By about five or six years old, many children can give a really good massage. They enjoy the percussion movements because they make such a lovely noise, the kneading because it is like playing with Plasticine, and the stroking because it is so easy. Above all, it's great fun.

IT'S EASY *for your child to massage your back if he sits or kneels on it. Just the pressure of his body alone can feel wonderful, particularly on the lower back.*

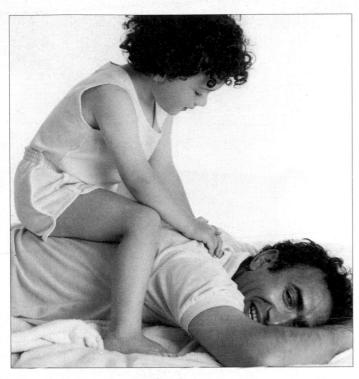

Kneading comes readily to a young child as it's just like playing with modelling clay. The vigorous movement is also an excellent way to burn up excess energy! Encourage your child to work on your shoulders and thighs.

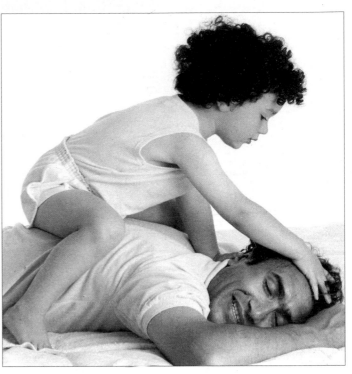

Let your child massage your face and forehead. Particularly after a hard day, a child's light touch can help to dispel tiredness and irritability, and generally make you feel better.

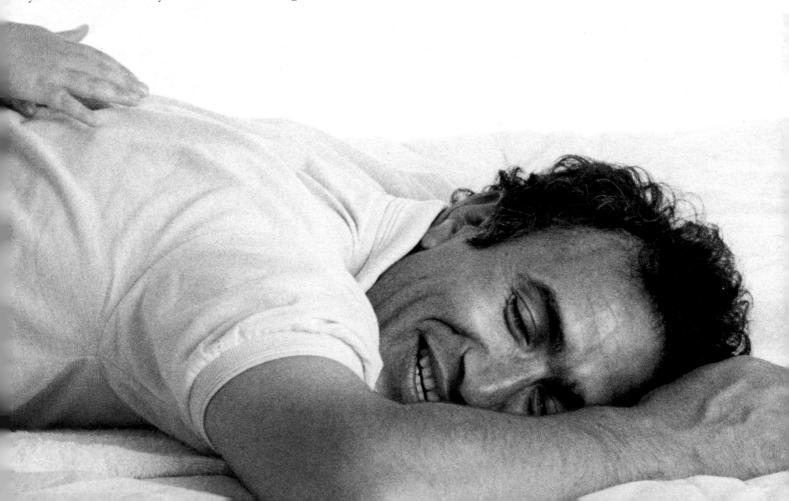

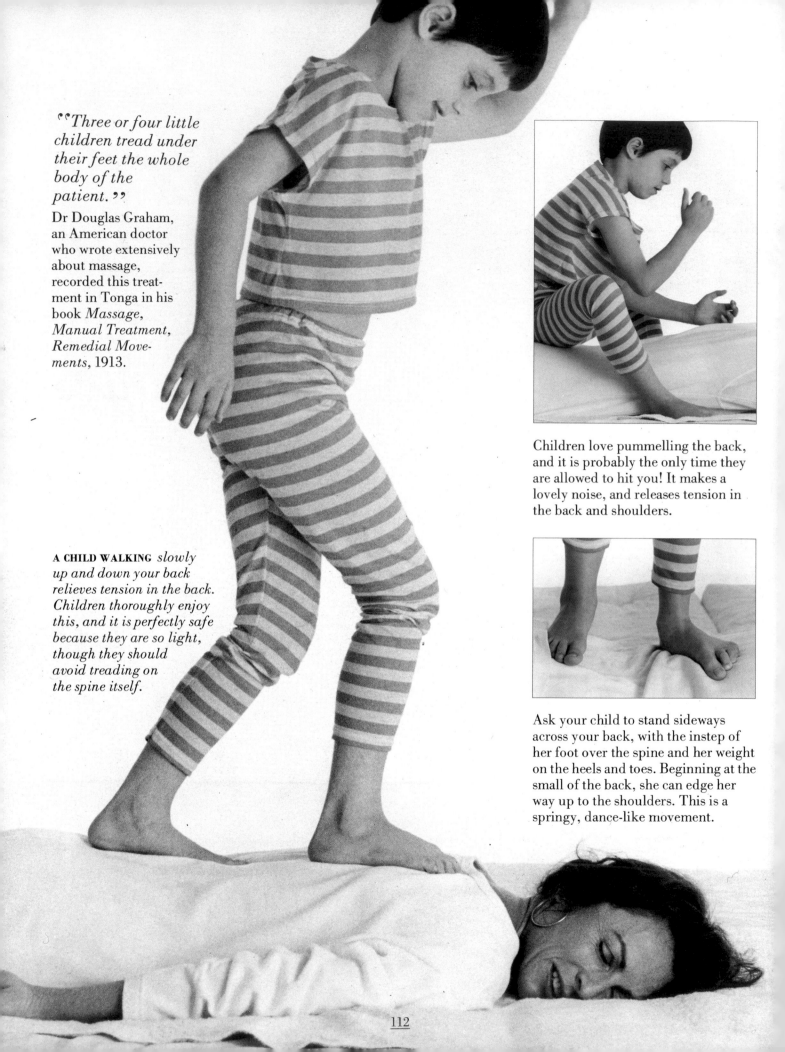

"Three or four little children tread under their feet the whole body of the patient."
Dr Douglas Graham, an American doctor who wrote extensively about massage, recorded this treatment in Tonga in his book *Massage, Manual Treatment, Remedial Movements*, 1913.

A CHILD WALKING *slowly up and down your back relieves tension in the back. Children thoroughly enjoy this, and it is perfectly safe because they are so light, though they should avoid treading on the spine itself.*

Children love pummelling the back, and it is probably the only time they are allowed to hit you! It makes a lovely noise, and releases tension in the back and shoulders.

Ask your child to stand sideways across your back, with the instep of her foot over the spine and her weight on the heels and toes. Beginning at the small of the back, she can edge her way up to the shoulders. This is a springy, dance-like movement.

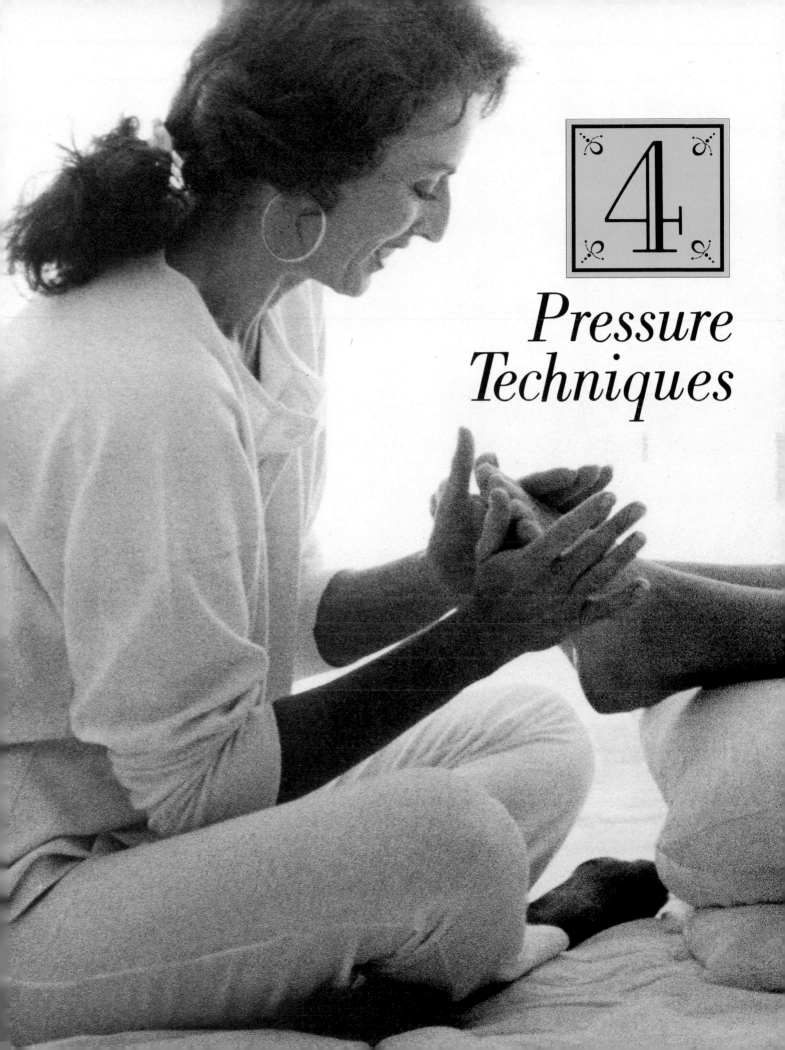

4

Pressure Techniques

SHIATSU

This oriental therapy, also known as acu-pressure, is a system of treating disorders by pressing firmly on the skin at precisely located points. It is based on the theory that the energy of life, known as chi, flows through the body along clearly defined channels which are called meridians. There are 14 main meridians, each of which influences a major organ of the body and any related organs and functions, although its path need not run close to the organ it is associated with. So, for example, the Lung meridian, which runs from the shoulder down to the thumb, influences the lungs and the entire breathing apparatus, including the nose and throat.

In a healthy person, the energy flows smoothly, and is balanced between the two oppo-site qualities, yin and yang. Yin is characterized as dark, cold and passive, while yang is seen as light, warm and active. The main meridians are grouped in pairs, one yin and one yang meridian in each pair. The yin meridians are on the inside or front surfaces of the body and the energy flows upwards, while the yang meridians are on the outside and back surfaces and the chi flows down-wards. If the flow of energy along a meridian is disrupted, the associated organ does not function properly and the person becomes unwell.

At a number of places along each meridian there are points where the energy can be contacted in order to restore a smooth and balanced flow through the channels. Shiatsu is the practice of treating these points by pressing on the skin.

Shiatsu is helpful in a wide variety of disorders, because by restoring energy balance in the body, it enables the body's own healing mechanisms to take over and cure the illness. When you become familiar with the concept of meridians, you can understand how different parts of the body are interrelated. I imagine the meridians as motor-ways running through the body, and with this image in mind it is easy to understand how tension or soreness in one area can be a signal that there is a problem elsewhere on the same meridian.

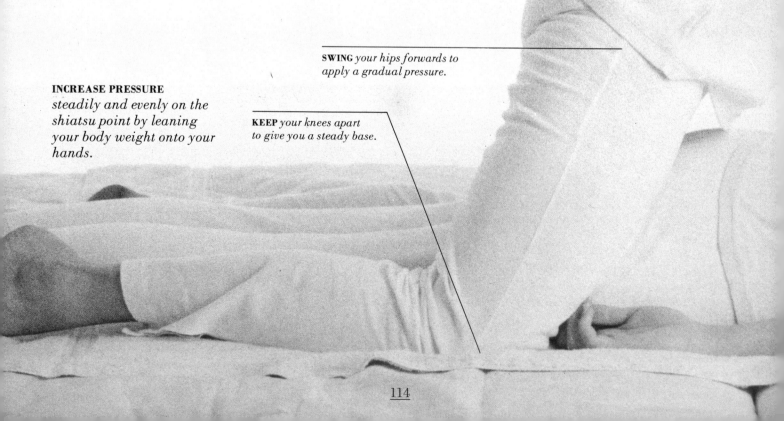

SWING *your hips forwards to apply a gradual pressure.*

INCREASE PRESSURE
steadily and evenly on the shiatsu point by leaning your body weight onto your hands.

KEEP *your knees apart to give you a steady base.*

LET THE PRESSURE *come from your shoulders.*

APPLYING PRESSURE

It is important to apply pressure correctly on the shiatsu points: you should build it up steadily, by gradually leaning your weight onto the point. Although it is usual to press with your thumbs, you can also use your fingers, the palms or heels of your hands and even your elbows (see page 119). The way you use your body is crucial to the treatment: keep your arms straight and slowly bring your shoulders over the point, swinging your hips forwards so that you gradually increase the pressure. With this technique, your pressure will be steady and even. If you use your body correctly, even the strongest of pressures should feel comfortable to the receiver, and you will avoid prodding or poking. On more delicate areas, such as the abdomen and face, you should still apply pressure steadily and evenly, but do not lean your full body weight onto the point.

At my courses, the students spend their first five minutes crawling around the room on their hands and knees. This is a simple way of teaching them how to relax their weight onto their hands, which is the key to applying pressure correctly in shiatsu.

KEEP *your arms straight.*

REST *your fingers lightly on the back.*

PRESS *with the ball of your thumbs.*

SHIATSU POINTS

Although there are about 600 shiatsu points on the body, I have shown only the key ones on the following pages. The points are positioned symmetrically, with corresponding points on the left and right hand sides of the body. Most points are given the name of the meridian they are on (usually the name of a major organ of the body), and a number to identify them. A few are called "extra points". You can use the points individually to alleviate minor ailments, or work systematically on the whole body to promote general health.

The points are quite easy to locate, and the body often helps you by having a slight indentation there. The measurements are given in finger widths, and it is best to measure with the fingers of the person you are massaging. The point is usually more sensitive than the surrounding area. When you press on it, the sensation seems to travel beyond that spot.

FRONT OF THE BODY

1 In the grooves between the ribs (points affecting the lungs).
2 End of the deltoid muscle (Large intestine 14).
3 On the forearm muscle, three finger widths below the elbow crease (Large intestine 10).
4 On the outside of the shin bone; measure the width across the knuckles below the knee (Stomach 36).
5 Down the centre of the abdomen; five finger widths and one finger width above the navel, and three finger widths below the navel (Conception vessel 12, 9 and 6). Press gently.
6 On the web of skin between the thumb and the index finger (Large intestine 4). Do not use this point on a pregnant woman, since it could cause miscarriage.
7 Find the spot where the middle finger touches the outer thigh when standing upright (Gall bladder 31).
8 In the groove behind the shin bone, four finger widths above the inside ankle prominence (Spleen 6).

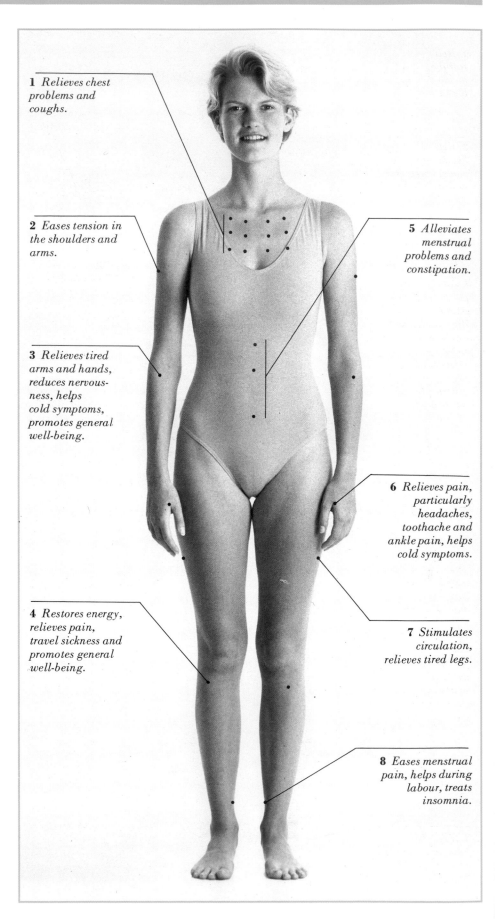

1 *Relieves chest problems and coughs.*

2 *Eases tension in the shoulders and arms.*

3 *Relieves tired arms and hands, reduces nervousness, helps cold symptoms, promotes general well-being.*

4 *Restores energy, relieves pain, travel sickness and promotes general well-being.*

5 *Alleviates menstrual problems and constipation.*

6 *Relieves pain, particularly headaches, toothache and ankle pain, helps cold symptoms.*

7 *Stimulates circulation, relieves tired legs.*

8 *Eases menstrual pain, helps during labour, treats insomnia.*

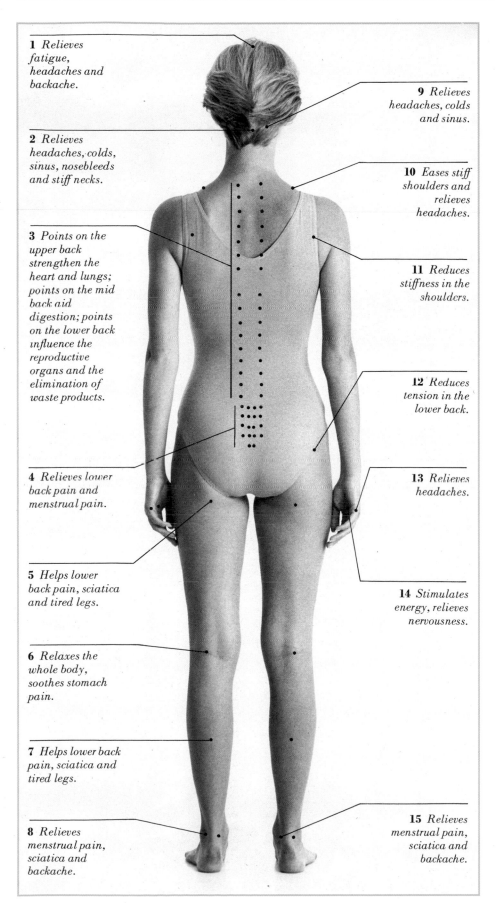

1 *Relieves fatigue, headaches and backache.*

2 *Relieves headaches, colds, sinus, nosebleeds and stiff necks.*

3 *Points on the upper back strengthen the heart and lungs; points on the mid back aid digestion; points on the lower back influence the reproductive organs and the elimination of waste products.*

4 *Relieves lower back pain and menstrual pain.*

5 *Helps lower back pain, sciatica and tired legs.*

6 *Relaxes the whole body, soothes stomach pain.*

7 *Helps lower back pain, sciatica and tired legs.*

8 *Relieves menstrual pain, sciatica and backache.*

9 *Relieves headaches, colds and sinus.*

10 *Eases stiff shoulders and relieves headaches.*

11 *Reduces stiffness in the shoulders.*

12 *Reduces tension in the lower back.*

13 *Relieves headaches.*

14 *Stimulates energy, relieves nervousness.*

15 *Relieves menstrual pain, sciatica and backache.*

BACK OF THE BODY

1 Crown of the head (Governing vessel 20).

2 Indentation in the base of the skull at the top of the neck (Governing vessel 15). Press up almost as though you were going under the skull.

3 On the muscles running down either side of the spine (Bladder 11 to 26).

4 On the sacrum (Bladder 27 to 35).

5 Centre of the back of the leg, directly under the buttock (Bladder 36).

6 Centre of the crease at the back of the knee (Bladder 40). Press gently, don't push the knee into the floor.

7 The middle of the calf muscle (Bladder 57).

8 On the outside of the ankle, between the ankle prominence and the Achilles tendon (Bladder 60).

9 Indentations in the base of the skull to either side of the spine (Gall bladder 20).

10 Centre of the muscle at the top of the shoulder (Gall bladder 21).

11 Slight indentation in the centre of the shoulder blade (Small intestine 11).

12 On the buttocks, just behind the hip joint (Gall bladder 30).

13 On the crease below the little finger, on the outside edge of the hand (Extra point).

14 Centre of the palm (Heart protector 8).

15 On the inside of the ankle, between the ankle prominence and the Achilles tendon (Kidney 3).

FACE

1 Points in a line from the centre of the hairline to the crown of the head (Governing vessel 21 to 24).
2 Small indentation on top of the centre of the eyebrow (Extra point).
3 On the top edge of the cheekbone, directly below the pupil of the eye when looking straight ahead (Stomach 1).
4 In the centre of the groove between the nose and the upper lip (Governing vessel 26).
5 Between the eyebrows (Extra point).
6 Inside corner of the eyes (Bladder 1).
7 Below the end of the eyebrow and level with the corner of the eye (Gall bladder 1).
8 Small groove at the side of the nose (Large intestine 20).

FEET

1 At the base of the big toe, between the big and second toes (Liver 2).
2 Lines of three pressures on the top of each toe (Extra points).
3 Two finger widths above point 1 (Liver 3).
4 On the outside of the little toe, at the base of the nail (Bladder 67).
5 On the centre of the sole, just below the ball of the foot (Kidney 1).

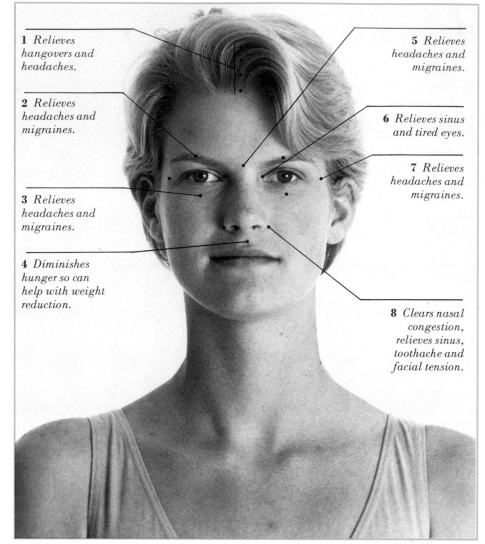

1 *Relieves hangovers and headaches.*
2 *Relieves headaches and migraines.*
3 *Relieves headaches and migraines.*
4 *Diminishes hunger so can help with weight reduction.*
5 *Relieves headaches and migraines.*
6 *Relieves sinus and tired eyes.*
7 *Relieves headaches and migraines.*
8 *Clears nasal congestion, relieves sinus, toothache and facial tension.*

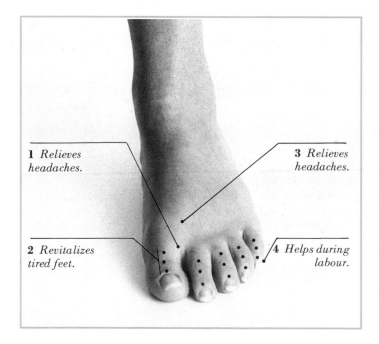

1 *Relieves headaches.*
2 *Revitalizes tired feet.*
3 *Relieves headaches.*
4 *Helps during labour.*

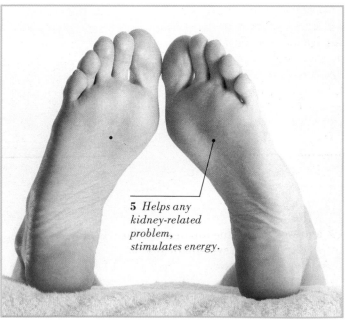

5 *Helps any kidney-related problem, stimulates energy.*

PRACTISING SHIATSU

Shiatsu treatments are always given on the floor, and your friend does not need to undress. Ask her to lie face down on a towel on the floor, then kneel by her side. Work systematically along the meridians, moving rhythmically from one point to the next. Press on the point as your friend breathes out, and hold for between three and seven seconds. Release the pressure as she breathes in, and move on. Always keep both hands on the body. If you are working with only one hand, rest the other gently on the body.

When you are familiar with the points, it will be second nature to use them during a massage. So, for example, when you are massaging the back, do firm pressures on the points running down either side of the spine.

The most effective way of using shiatsu is to treat the whole body, to harmonize energy, which takes about 45 minutes to an hour. The sequence below is a simplified and shortened version, which will improve the circulation and induce relaxation.

1 Press down either side of the spine. Use the heels of your hands first, then repeat with your thumbs.

2 Press down the buttocks and the back of the legs, keeping the pressure light over the knees.

3 Ask your friend to turn over, and squeeze down the arms, pressing on the points on the arms and hands.

4 Apply pressures down the front of the legs and the feet, but avoid pressing hard on the knees.

5 Press gently with your palm on the abdomen, working clockwise in a large circle.

6 Kneel behind your friend's head and work from the top of the head down over the face, systematically pressing on all the points.

7 Work from the centre of the chest outwards, pressing in lines between the ribs.

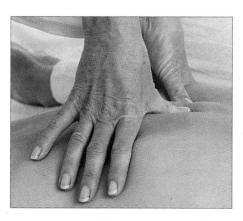

USE THE BALL of your thumb and rest your fingers on the skin to help you give a steady, even pressure. Do not use the tip of your thumb, because your nail, however short, will gouge the skin. Work with both thumbs at the same time or one at a time.

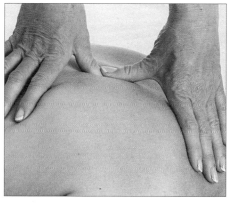

FOR EXTRA DEPTH on the shoulders, buttocks, back and soles of the feet, put one thumb on top of the other.

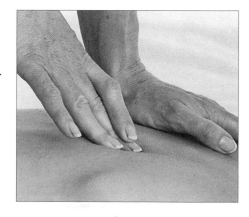

IF YOU USE your fingers, put your index finger on top of your middle finger for more depth. This is useful if your thumbs are tired or sore.

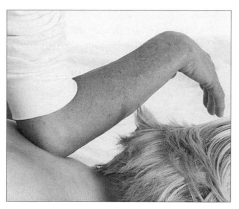

IF YOU USE your elbow, make sure that your arm and hand are relaxed so that you apply a gentle pressure, not a hard prod. This is useful on large muscular areas such as the shoulder muscle, the buttocks and the back of the thighs.

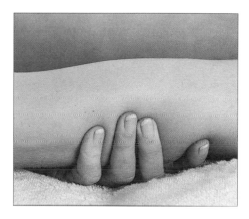

TREAT SMALLER AREAS such as the arms by squeezing them between the thumb and fingers.

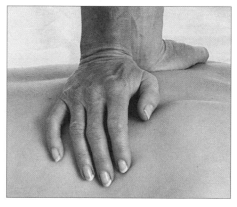

USE THE HEEL of your hand to give a more general stimulation to the point. This technique is most often used on the back or the legs.

REFLEXOLOGY

This therapy focuses on stimulating reflex points on the feet to maintain good health. It is based on the theory that every part of the body corresponds to a very precisely located point on the feet, and that by applying pressure to these reflex points, you can relax and balance the whole body and help treat a range of disorders. Thus, for example, stomach problems can be treated by pressure just below the ball of the foot, and headaches by pressure on the big toe. Most of the reflex points are on the soles of the feet, but there are some on the top and round the ankles.

According to reflexologists, a disorder in any part of the body is reflected by sensitivity in the corresponding area of the feet. Reflexologists do not claim to diagnose illness, but a good therapist can usually tell where there is a weakness in the body. Clients are frequently amazed at the accuracy of reflexology in pinpointing some detail about the state of their health.

The feet are a very complex structure, and foot problems can result in postural and other disorders. Corns and callouses may cause problems in the corresponding parts of the body. It is extraordinary how often people with lung problems have callouses on the balls of their feet (the area corresponding to the lungs), and people with bunions have neck problems.

Although there is no scientific explanation of how reflexology works, the therapy is very successful. At the very least, massaging the feet in this way is incredibly relaxing, and this has general beneficial effects on health. Tense muscles reduce their restrictive grip on blood vessels, thus enabling blood to circulate freely, distributing nutrients to the cells and removing waste products. In addition, a reflexology treatment can improve many foot problems.

Hand reflexology
There are similar reflex points on the hands but, since they are deeper, they are less sensitive and more difficult to locate than those on the feet. However, this is balanced by the fact that most people love having their hands worked on and find it very relaxing, and hand reflexology is easy to practise anywhere. The reflex points are in much the same places as on the feet: most are located on the palms, with the fingers and thumbs corresponding to the head.

History of reflexology
Reflexology as we know it today grew out of Eunice Ingham's work with zone therapy (see below) in the 1930s. A medical masseuse, she found that she could treat the entire body by applying pressure to the feet, and her treatments proved tremendously successful. She developed a map on the feet to show the location of reflex points for every part of the body, and this map forms the basis for reflexology.

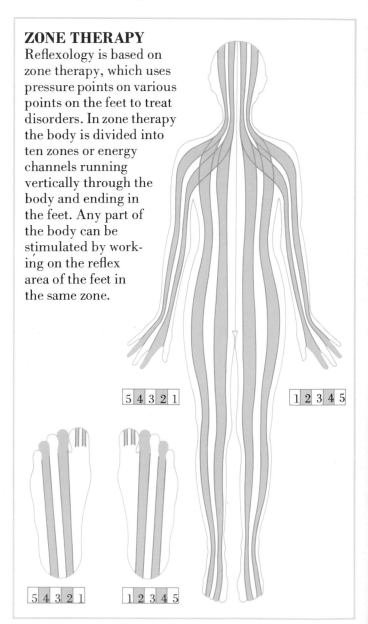

ZONE THERAPY
Reflexology is based on zone therapy, which uses pressure points on various points on the feet to treat disorders. In zone therapy the body is divided into ten zones or energy channels running vertically through the body and ending in the feet. Any part of the body can be stimulated by working on the reflex area of the feet in the same zone.

REFLEX POINTS

An easy way of remembering the location of the reflex points is to visualize a picture of the body superimposed on the soles of the feet. The big toe corresponds to the head, the inside edges of the feet correspond to the spine, and the reflexes for the main organs are located roughly according to their position in the body.

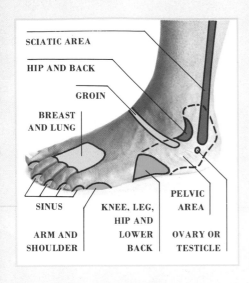

SCIATIC AREA
HIP AND BACK
GROIN
BREAST AND LUNG
SINUS
KNEE, LEG, HIP AND LOWER BACK
ARM AND SHOULDER
PELVIC AREA
OVARY OR TESTICLE

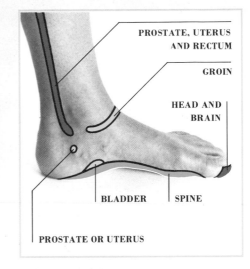

PROSTATE, UTERUS AND RECTUM
GROIN
HEAD AND BRAIN
BLADDER
SPINE
PROSTATE OR UTERUS

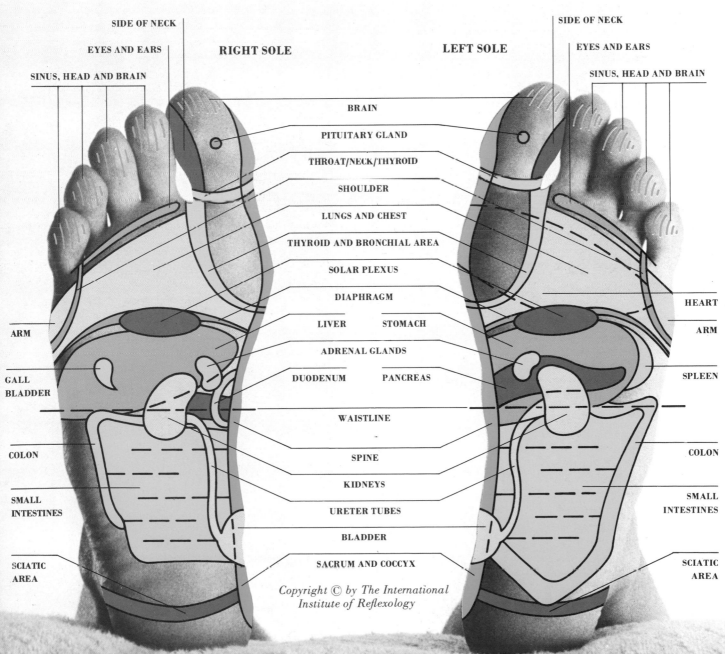

RIGHT SOLE **LEFT SOLE**

SIDE OF NECK
EYES AND EARS
SINUS, HEAD AND BRAIN

BRAIN
PITUITARY GLAND
THROAT/NECK/THYROID
SHOULDER
LUNGS AND CHEST
THYROID AND BRONCHIAL AREA
SOLAR PLEXUS
DIAPHRAGM
HEART
LIVER   STOMACH
ARM
ADRENAL GLANDS
SPLEEN
DUODENUM   PANCREAS
GALL BLADDER
WAISTLINE
COLON
SPINE
COLON
KIDNEYS
SMALL INTESTINES
URETER TUBES
SMALL INTESTINES
BLADDER
SCIATIC AREA
SACRUM AND COCCYX
SCIATIC AREA

ARM

Copyright © by The International Institute of Reflexology

PRACTISING REFLEXOLOGY

During a reflexology session, your friend should sit comfortably with her legs supported and a cushion under her knees. Some reflexologists treat their clients lying down, but I prefer being able to see the face of the person I am treating, so that I can tell whether an area of the foot is sensitive, and can maintain eye contact. Sit or kneel at your friend's feet and place them in your lap or rest them on a stool. Work over the whole foot to promote and maintain good health. As you work, you may come across sensitive areas which indicate a problem in the corresponding part of the body. In some places it even feels as if there are granules under the skin. Give extra attention to these areas to disperse the granules in the feet and reduce congestion elsewhere. In this way you can treat a variety of complaints from headaches and backache to digestive problems and insomnia. Pressures on these areas may be rather painful, so watch your friend's face to make sure you are not hurting her. It is better to treat a disorder by working gently and repeating the treatment several times, rather than overworking sensitive areas in the hope of treating disorders all in one go.

TECHNIQUE

Do not massage the feet, simply apply a precise pressure with your thumb to each specific point. Hold the foot firmly with one hand, and work with the other thumb, using the edge of the thumb, just by the nail. Press firmly for about three seconds, then move on with an inching forwards movement. Do not use oil, since this will make your thumbs slip; lightly dust the feet with talcum powder or work directly on the skin.

A complete reflexology treatment takes about 45 minutes to 1 hour. The following sequence is simply a short introduction to reflexology. Treat the right foot first, then the left foot.

HOLD *the foot firmly with one hand.*

PRESS FIRMLY *with the edge of your thumb, just by the nail.*

PASSIVE MOVEMENTS

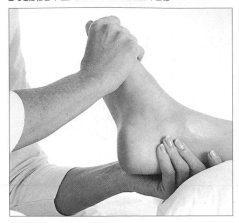 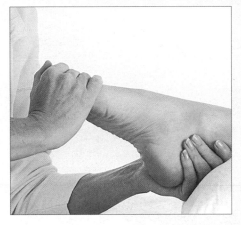 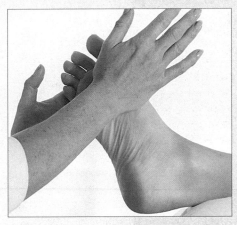

1 Start your treatment by relaxing the foot with some passive movements. Support and stabilize the ankle with one hand, and hold the toes firmly with your other hand. Rotate the foot four times in each direction.

2 Keep one hand under the ankle and the other holding the toes. Stretch the foot slowly back and forth to release tension in the Achilles tendon. Never force the joint further than it will comfortably go.

3 Loosen and warm the whole foot by rolling it quickly from side to side between your palms.

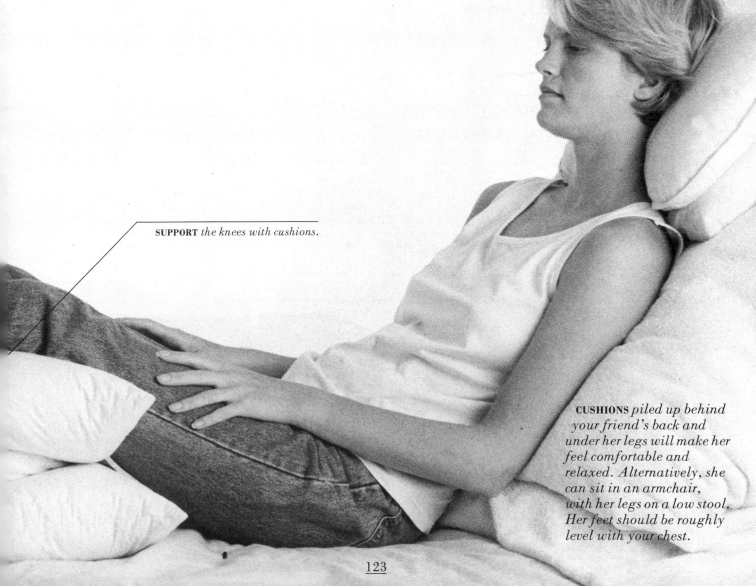

SUPPORT *the knees with cushions.*

CUSHIONS *piled up behind your friend's back and under her legs will make her feel comfortable and relaxed. Alternatively, she can sit in an armchair, with her legs on a low stool. Her feet should be roughly level with your chest.*

BASIC SEQUENCE

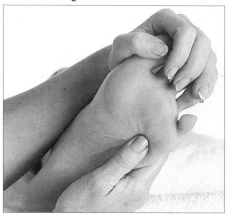

1 Press along the diaphragm line under the ball of the foot. Then stimulate the spinal area by working from the heel along the main arch of the foot to the big toe.

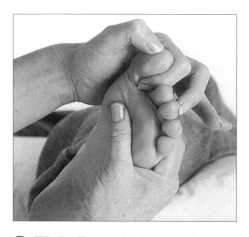

2 Work all over the big toe. Cover the area thoroughly, since it corresponds to the head. Then work on the back, sides and top of each of the other toes.

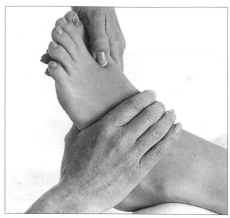

3 Apply a line of pressures between the tendons on the top of the foot. Work from the base of the toes to the ankle in each furrow. This releases tension in the chest and breast.

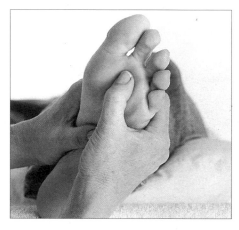

4 Apply pressures all over the ball of the foot underneath the big toe, to treat the lungs. On the left foot, pay extra attention to the heart area towards the inside edge.

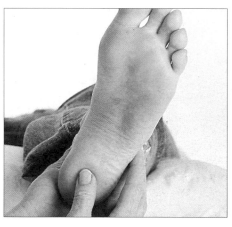

5 Do pressures in diagonal lines, working from the waist line to the diaphragm line. Then work in the same way from the heel to the waist line to treat the digestive system.

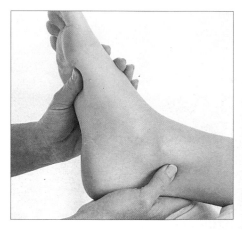

6 Apply pressures all round the ankle. This area corresponds to the lower back, reproductive organs and legs. Then work all over the heel to prevent or treat lower back pain.

SELF-REFLEXOLOGY
Although it is inevitably a little less relaxing than receiving a treatment from someone else, it is quite possible to give yourself an effective reflexology treatment.

Reflexologists recommend that you work on your feet each day to promote health. A healthy body is reflected in healthy, pain-free feet, so you should start looking after your feet today.

Either sit comfortably with one foot resting on the thigh of the opposite leg, or lie down with one leg bent, and rest the opposite foot on your raised thigh. Slowly explore the whole foot, following the sequence given above. Pay extra attention to any sore or sensitive areas: build up pressure on them gradually, and return to work on them several times, trying to dispel the soreness.

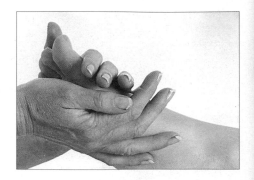

7 Finish by stroking the foot gently from the ankle to the toes, to soothe the whole area.

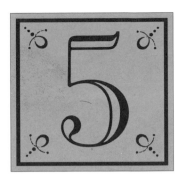

Therapeutic Massage

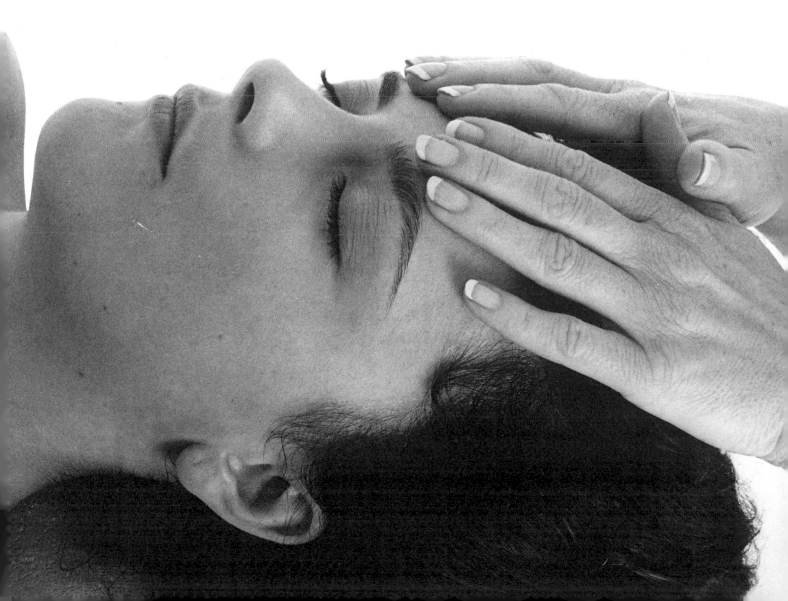

THE HEALING POWER OF MASSAGE

Massage has a long tradition as a healing therapy and has been used by many cultures for centuries to treat and alleviate a wide range of disorders. Dr Stretch Dowse, an eminent Victorian doctor, wrote in 1887: "It seems to me that massage is destined to play a very important part in the future of the human race". He even went so far as to liken its benefits for the human body to the role of engineering in sanitation, observing that "the present system of drainage, if effectually carried out, keeps a house healthy and pure. The system of massage, if properly conducted, tends to maintain the pure mind in the healthy body."

A truly complementary therapy, massage is a positive way of comforting someone who is ill and relieving unpleasant symptoms. By stroking and soothing you are helping a patient to relax and improving the quality of his rest and sleep. The simple act of touching can play an indispensable part in the healing process. The immune system, which helps the body to fight disease, is stimulated when the patient feels cared for: the sheer pleasure of massage is therapeutic.

If your friend is seriously ill, do not massage without his doctor's consent. Never massage anyone suffering from any of the following conditions, since massage could spread an infection or irritate an inflamed area:
- an infectious disease
- a high temperature
- a skin infection
- an inflammatory condition such as thrombosis or phlebitis.

Bear in mind that you can relax the whole body by massaging just a few areas. Next time you visit a friend in hospital, why not give him a hand massage? As a hospital visitor, it can be difficult thinking of ways to entertain the patient, and all too often the patient becomes exhausted from entertaining the visitor. It is far easier for you, and more relaxing for your friend, if you give him a massage.

When you are massaging someone who is ill, take extra care to make sure that he is warm and comfortable. Use lots of soothing, gentle stroking movements and remember that even the simplest massage will be greatly appreciated.

MANUAL LYMPH DRAINAGE

The lymphatic system, which acts as a purifying and drainage system for the body (see page 141), is put under strain when the body is injured or unhealthy. Waste products cannot be filtered out quickly enough and build up, causing swelling at the site of injury or around the lymph nodes.

Manual lymph drainage is a gentle, pumping massage which aims to speed up the removal of waste products by stimulating the lymphatic system. The technique is very useful on anyone with swelling or any injury, particularly a sports injury. Fluid retention may be relieved, and even acne and eczema may improve.

All the movements are performed up the body towards the nearest lymph nodes, starting nearest the body and moving out to the extremities. The main lymph nodes are in the neck, armpits, groin, behind the knees and on the inside of the elbows.

Since the lymph vessels are close to the surface, your pressure should be very light. It is hard to believe that something so gentle could be so effective, but the following passage written by J.B. Memmel, a physiotherapist, in 1945 demonstrates the success of such a light massage on a swollen ankle: "An officer had been receiving massage treatments for many weeks before he came under my care. He at first laughed at the idea that our gentle handling could help him, when his former vigorous treatments had failed to do so. In a week he had changed his mind on finding the circumference of his ankle reduced by over 12 inches from the size it had been for many weeks. He added that he had thought I was crazy when I first ordered massage to begin on the thigh, when his trouble was in his foot."

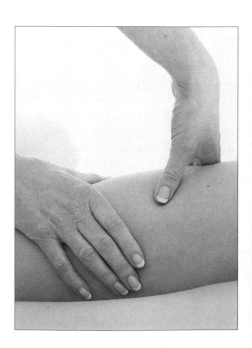

MANUAL LYMPH DRAINAGE *is an extremely soft, rhythmic and monotonous form of massage. I find it helps if I visualize that I am pumping the fluid up to the lymph nodes.*

GRATEFUL PAIN

"The finger of a good rubber will descend upon a painful nerve as gently as dew on grass, and upon a torrid callosity as heavily as the hoof of an elephant." (Beveridge, a Scottish masseur, 1774-1839).

When doing a massage you will almost inevitably come across tender points on the body that seem to be asking to be pressed. If you press on these points, it may be painful at first, but it is usually the "Ooh that's wonderful" type of pain, or as one of my clients calls it, "grateful pain". Pressure on these points can have a profound effect: it can relieve tension, release taut muscles and eradicate pain.

Press on a point gently at first and, as your friend breathes out, build up pressure by leaning your body weight onto the point, using your thumbs, fingers or elbows. Hold the pressure for about three to seven seconds, then release it gently.

It is not a question of crushing the tissue as you press, but of finding the target. Your friend will be able to tell you whether you have found one of the right points: he should feel "grateful pain", not just ordinary pain. I know this sounds confusing, but when you experience the right sort of pain you will understand what it is.

Watch your friend's reaction very carefully as you apply the pressure. Although the area is sensitive, your pressure should not feel painful. If your friend winces, or if you feel a muscle tightening up, decrease your pressure slightly. You can always return to the spot later on. If it is very tender, stroke the surrounding area gently to reduce muscle spasm before pressing on the point.

A case where deep pressure of this sort successfully treated a painful attack of arthritis is reported by the Victorian physician Dr Cornelius in a book written in 1909. A man suffering from this condition was given a daily massage. He noticed that one physician, who sought out and concentrated on the painful areas, was much more successful than the others. He wrote: "Stimulated by this, I also palpated my sore regions and found that most of them were painless, but that there were a few regions without regular distribution, which were sensitive to the gentlest touch. I then asked my masseurs to treat only those regions which I had discovered to be painful instead of giving the general massage. The success was astonishing: swelling as well as pain disappeared in a very short time, and while previously I had not experienced the least improvement, ∴ after four weeks of this kind of massage I was free of swelling and complaints, and was able to return to duty apparently recovered, feeling strong and healthy."

STRESS

"The mind, which before massage is in a perturbed, restless, vacillating and even despondent state, becomes after massage, calm, quiet, peaceful and subdued; in fact, the wearied and worried mind has been converted into a mind restful, placid and refreshed," wrote the Victorian doctor, Stretch Dowse, in 1887.

Although a certain amount of stress is essential to add zest to life, too much stress has negative effects. There is a strong link between stress and illness. Many doctors notice that their patients are less resistant to disease after an emotionally stressful event. High blood pressure and heart disease are related to stress. Other disorders such as cancer, rheumatism, headaches, backache, acne, infertility and even infectious diseases are all more likely to develop when resistance is low.

Massage is the ideal way of reducing stress, whether physical or emotional. By relaxing taut muscles, it enables the whole body and mind to relax.

When treating patients at the Kaiser-Permanente Medical Center in San José, California, Dr David Sobel, Chief of Preventive Medicine, observed that what many of his patients really needed was to be touched. "My sense is that many of these people would be much more helped by a skilful massage than the usual ministrations of doctors. One of the greatest problems facing many of us is that we have become so accustomed to tension, that we don't know what it feels like to be really relaxed. How often I hear patients with hunched, tense shoulders and clenched jaws say: 'But I am relaxed'. A massage offers not only immediate pleasure and relief, but the opportunity to glimpse deeper relaxation. By definition this can improve our health and massage should certainly be considered a valuable resource in therapy as well as health promotion. Those who would think otherwise have probably never had a good massage."

USING MASSAGE

If you are trying to help someone who is suffering from stress, follow the basic massage sequence given in Chapter 1 (see pages 22 to 79), concentrating on whatever areas your friend likes best. Keep the whole massage rhythmic and flowing. Mix some of the essential oils listed on page 20 with your massage oil, choosing ones that will enhance the relaxing effect of the massage.

I have numerous clients who, through regular massage, have stopped using tranquillizers or seeing their psychiatrists. Massage is the very best tranquillizer – just as effective as drugs or alcohol, and so much better for you.

INSOMNIA

"In insomnia general massage at bed-time undoubtedly promotes sleep. The result is not only certain but prompt, the patient usually enjoying a good night's rest after the first seance. It has the advantage over all narcotics that there are no disagreeable side effects." (William Murrel M.D. F.R.C.P. *Massotherapeutics*, 1889).

One of the most satisfying things about massage is its ability to send someone to sleep. It is so rewarding to watch someone drift off and then to creep away leaving him fast asleep. Even if it takes a little while, you will find that the soothing and hypnotic strokes of massage nearly always work their magic.

Massage is an ideal remedy for insomnia. Sleeping pills are not the answer: although they can be useful in a crisis, continued use can be habit-forming, and if they are taken regularly, they lose their effectiveness. Massage becomes more effective the more often it is used, and gives a deep, natural sleep without any after-effects in the morning.

I have numerous clients who used to suffer from insomnia, and have been able to break the habit with the help of relaxation and massage. A doctor recently sent an eleven-year-old girl and her mother to me to learn massage. Both were very tense and nervous, and the daughter suffered from insomnia. I taught the mother how to massage her daughter. This not only helped the girl to sleep, but also calmed the mother. That is the wonderful thing about massage, it works both ways and can be of equal benefit to the giver and the receiver.

GIVING A MASSAGE

If you are trying to cure someone's habit of insomnia, you should give him a massage regularly at bed time until you have broken the habit. Your friend should lie in his bed, so that if he falls asleep while you are massaging, you can leave him to sleep.

Some people have great difficulty relaxing: if your friend does not fall asleep the first time you massage, don't give up. Persevere, and maybe next time your hypnotic strokes will work. Most people, though, respond quickly, so your friend will probably doze off almost instantly. If so, don't stop massaging immediately – your strokes will enhance his sleep. Continue massaging in time to his breathing until you have finished, then creep away, leaving him asleep.

When trying to send someone to sleep, you should ideally do a complete body, face and head massage, which takes about 1½ hours. If you do not have that much time, you will get the quickest results by concentrating on the back, abdomen, feet and face. You can massage all four areas, or just one, depending on how quickly your friend relaxes. The order of the massage does not matter – just follow your friend's preference. Keep all your movements smooth, rhythmic and hypnotic.

Back

Place one hand on the nape of the neck and the other on the small of the back. Hold your hands there for about 30 seconds and breathe deeply and slowly. This encourages your friend to breathe deeply himself and to focus attention on any tense areas. Then start massaging: follow the basic massage sequence for the back, but

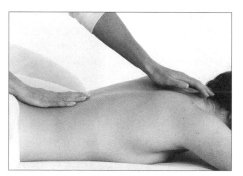

THE CAT STROKE *is very soporific. Glide your hands slowly down the back, one after the other. After a few minutes of this, your friend should be fast asleep.*

miss out any stimulating movements such as pummelling, and spend a long time on soothing strokes such as the cat stroke. Massage fairly firmly at first and, as you see your friend relax, work more and more softly.

Abdomen, feet and face

Give a very gentle, smooth massage on each area, using lots of rhythmic stroking. The final touch should be extremely slow and sensitive, and you can repeat it several times.

SHIATSU TREATMENT

A Chinese friend of mine had been dependent on sleeping pills for thirty years when she decided to stop using them and find another solution to her sleep problem. She tried shiatsu, and was amazed at her success. The treatment is simple, takes only about ten minutes, and you can easily treat yourself.

My friend began by doing shiatsu every two hours for a couple of days, then just in the morning and evening. Although she had expected to use shiatsu rather like sleeping pills, with doses every day, after a few months she no longer needed shiatsu to sleep. She had been thinking in terms of Western medicine, whereas in Oriental medicine, once you have unblocked the chi (the energy of life that flows through the meridians) and it is circulating correctly, your symptoms go and you are cured of the disorder.

If you suffer from severe insomnia, treat yourself frequently at first, then decrease the number of treatments. If you have a sleepless night, use shiatsu a bit more frequently for a day or so. Sit comfortably at a table or on the floor, and wear loose clothing so that you can relax your stomach. Close your eyes and breathe deeply and evenly as you apply the pressures. Concentrate on the feeling of pressure. When you locate the exact points, they feel slightly tender, and you may get an expanding, releasing sensation. Sit quietly and relax for a few minutes after you finish.

HEADACHES AND MIGRAINE

Massage can be tremendously helpful in dispelling the headaches and migraines that plague so many of us. It is thought that most headaches are caused by changes in blood pressure in the blood vessels leading to and from the brain. When a muscle is in spasm, it squeezes and constricts the blood vessels, so relaxing the muscle allows blood to flow more freely, alleviating the headache. Even severe headaches can sometimes disappear after only a few minutes' massage.

The type of massage depends on the intensity of the headache, and what your friend prefers. You can use very gentle feather stroking or deep, firm pressure. It is generally best to start with slow, superficial stroking and then as the pain subsides and your friend relaxes and feels confident of your touch, you can apply firm pressures to key points.

The Victorian doctor, Stretch Dowse, observed that, when treating migraines, "with gentle stroking, a condition of hypnosis is induced, during which the pain disappears." Another Victorian, Dr Deyardin-Beaumetz, advocated a rather different treatment: "In cases of frontal headache or migraine the thumb or forefinger is pressed on the tender spot."

HEADACHE CURE
Although every headache is different, I find that I get the best results by following this general pattern. When you are treating a headache, all your movements should be very smooth, rhythmic and compassionate.

1 Stroke up the forehead very gently and slowly.

2 Stroke the chest and shoulders, then rhythmically stroke up the back of the neck.

3 Apply circular pressures behind the shoulders, up the neck on either side of the spine, and all around the base of the skull.

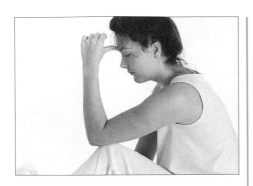

1 Press between your eyebrows (Extra point). Rest your elbow on your knee, and lean your weight onto your thumb. Hold the pressure for 10 to 15 seconds, then release.

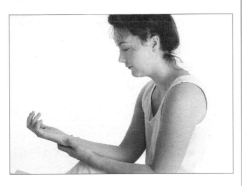

2 Press on the slight depression on the inside of your wrist, below your little finger (Heart 7). Press with your thumb, and support your wrist with your fingers. Hold the pressure for 10 to 15 seconds, then repeat on the other wrist.

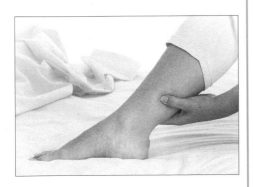

3 Measure four fingers' width up from the ankle bone on the inside of your ankle (Spleen 6). Rest your little finger on the bony prominence; the point is level with your index finger, behind the shin bone. Press with your thumb for seven to ten seconds on each ankle.

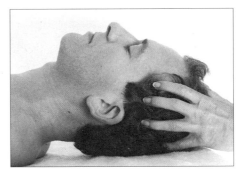

4 Continue these circular pressures over the scalp and round the ears.

5 Gently stroke the whole face from the centre out to the sides.

6 Press the bridge of the nose, then pinch the eyebrows and press on the temples.

7 Press in the middle of the cheek, directly under the cheekbone.

8 Apply a line of pressures up the centre of the forehead, from between the eyebrows to the hairline.

9 Circle round the eyes, stroking out along the eyebrows and gliding back gently under the eyes.

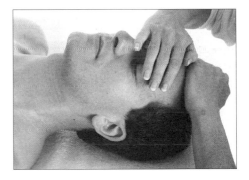

10 Stroke rhythmically up the forehead with one hand following the other, as you did at the beginning.

OTHER CURES
If there is very little time or I am treating a very severe migraine, I get the best results by imagining that my hands are magnets, drawing out all the tension and pain. For this, use the feather touch, stroking tension away from the head and off the body. Massaging firmly all round the base of your thumb can also help alleviate a migraine; try this simple remedy whenever you feel a headache or migraine coming on.

SHIATSU-BASED CURE FOR HEADACHE

I was taught this headache cure in Sarawak, and it really seems to work. It is easy to practise on yourself, but do not use the first shiatsu point if you are pregnant. Press on each point for between three and seven seconds.

1 *Pinch hard on the web of skin between your thumb and forefinger.*

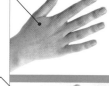

2 *Make your hand into a fist and pinch just below the little finger.*

3 *Press firmly on the back of the wrist in the middle.*

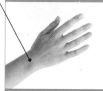

4 *Press in the middle of the forearm.*

5 *Bend your elbow, press on the middle of the outside.*

6 *Press on either side of the spine at the waist.*

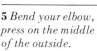

7 *Press at the bridge of the nose.*

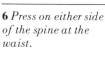

8 *Press in the middle of the eyebrows.*

9 *Stroke up the forehead from the bridge of the nose to the hair.*

10 *Apply circular pressures in lines out across the forehead.*

11 *Press and circle on the temples for about 30 seconds.*

12 *Press and circle above the ears and into the hair to cover the whole scalp.*

Shiatsu cure for migraine

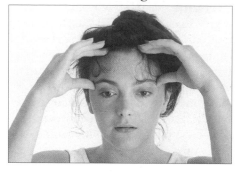

1 Press between the outer corner of the eye and the eyebrow (Gall bladder 1).

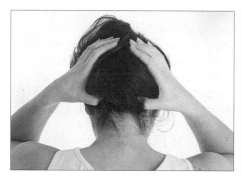

2 Press at the base of the skull and to either side (Bladder 10, Governing vessel 15).

3 Pinch the web of skin between the thumb and forefinger – see step 1, left (Large intestine 4).

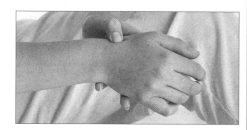

4 Press in the depression formed by the two tendons at the base of the thumb (Large intestine 5).

Shiatsu cure for sinus headache

1 Press in the middle of each eyebrow and between your eyebrows (Extra points).

2 Press on the cheekbones below the centre of your eyes (Stomach 1).

3 Pinch both sides of your hand just below the knuckle at the base of your little finger (Extra point).

BEREAVEMENT

Massage is a direct and powerful form of communication which can show care and provide comfort at times when words are inadequate. Bereavement is one such time, and the benefits of massage can be enormous. Bereaved people sometimes keep their emotions bottled up, and massage can work as a safety valve by releasing both physical and mental tension. By doing this, it can help them to recover from their grief more quickly.

This first came home to me some years ago when a client lost her 21-year-old son in a motor-bike accident, and another client lost his wife from a heart attack. Their lives were suddenly totally disrupted, and they suffered from shock and isolation. Normal communication seemed pointless, yet through massage I became close to them and gently helped both of them to return to ordinary life.

Friends and family may not recognize the need for touch, although physical contact can be greatly missed, particularly in someone who has been married for a long time. A widow whose husband had died three years earlier came to me for a massage to release tension in her neck and shoulders. As I massaged her, the tension seemed to melt away. She told me that her husband had been a physically affectionate man, and that she missed the warmth of human touch. After a few massages she slept better, regained her desire to live, and became more active and social.

You do not need to do a full body massage to show that you care. Simply stroke the bereaved person's hands, or massage his neck and shoulders.

HEART DISEASE

Heart disease is the leading cause of premature death in the Western world, and massage has an important part to play in the treatment of patients suffering from heart disease or recovering after a heart attack. Dr Peter Nixon, a consultant cardiologist at a London hospital, explains why: "The human body is in a constant state of arousal; receiving messages that accelerate or decelerate the body's nervous system. When the accelerator is down, chemical changes cascade through the body, activating the arousal mechanisms. The 'tread-mill' of arousal works all right when there is an equilibrium between effort, rest and sleep, but to maintain a healthy balance, we need other things. We need to feel that our efforts are worthwhile. We need 'strokes' of appreciation from others. If we don't get them, we more easily lose heart and our internal systems more easily fall into disarray. Immunity to disease is reduced and the body's internal functions are degraded. Homeostasis, the body's self-regulating system, cannot manage the internal house-keeping. It needs to be re-established and a healthy function recreated. This is where massage comes in. Good massage is marvellous for reducing arousal, producing a calm state and providing the opportunity for repair-ing the effects of wear and tear and overspending energy. The good masseur can create a relationship which shows the patient how to get well."

ANGINA

Massage can help to ease the vice-like crushing pain of angina and alleviate the feeling of isolation that accom-panies such a condition. But do be guided by the sufferer. Some people may not want to be touched at all during an attack, others may be soothed if you stroke their forehead or shoulders. A hand massage can divert attention from the pain and help to alleviate tension.

HEART ATTACKS AND HEART SURGERY

I give massage to heart attack patients regularly in the cardiac department of a hospital. During their recovery it is crucial for patients to relax and to keep their blood pressure down, to minimize the chances of a second heart attack. Most of them are tense and nervous, and a great many simply do not know how to relax, although they are utterly exhausted. Massage puts them into a state of deep relaxation, lowers blood pressure and helps them to sleep. A nurse measures the patient's blood pressure before and after the half-hour massage, and it nearly always falls. In some cases the drop has been dramatic, for example from 180/130 to 140/100 mmHg.

On one occasion I massaged a woman who had suffered from heart disease for many years. During her massage in the cardiac ward, she said: "This is the nearest thing to heaven one can get on this earth. Better than all the drugs I've had for the last 16 years." On another occasion I was asked to try to calm down a very tense, aggressive man. He was a most difficult patient, and seemed to hate everyone and everything. He only grudgingly agreed to let me give him a massage, but when I had finished he said: "Well, at least that's one thing worth living for."

The eminent Victorian cardiologist, Sir Lauder Brunton, observed that "in cases of cardiac disease, massage allows the other treatments to be carried out more easily than it would otherwise be, for it removes the feeling of weariness and irritability, fidgeti-ness and unrest. The appetite increases and the spirits become brighter."

If you are trying to help someone recover from a heart attack or after heart surgery, you must obtain his doctor's permission before you start. With the doctor's approval you can begin to massage as soon as the patient is out of the intensive care unit.

Follow the sequence given in Chapter 1, but massage a little more slowly than usual, and watch the patient carefully to make sure that he is enjoying the massage. All your movements must be very gentle and soothing, with firmer strokes moving towards the heart, and light strokes gliding away. After heart surgery, avoid the chest area altogether for a while, or massage it extremely gently, especially round the scar.

I usually give a gentle full body massage, concentrating on those areas where the patient feels most tense – often the back, shoulders, chest, head, feet and abdomen. It is just a question of calming and soothing the patient, so do whatever he finds most enjoyable and relaxing.

THERAPY OF GIVING

Besides giving a massage to patients, I also teach their partners to massage them. It is not always possible for the patients to continue having a professional massage, but if their partners know how to massage, it is always available, literally, at their fingertips.

I often notice, though, that the "well" partners are the ones most in need of the massage. They tend to be very tense and over-tired; they have to live with the anxiety of the illness, cope with the extra workload and, as everyone's sympathy is directed towards the patients, they frequently suffer from a lack of attention. If this condition continues for years, the "well" partners can become exhausted, depressed and even ill themselves.

I now try to teach both partners how to massage – and both benefit from this. The "well" partners' feelings of helplessness in the face of a serious illness are eased by providing comfort and help. The patients benefit from being able to give for a change. It can be difficult to be ill and always on the receiving end. Massage is an easy way of doing something for their partners and showing appreciation. This in turn is a great boost to their self-esteem, which can be sadly lacking after a long illness.

VARICOSE VEINS

These are permanently and unevenly dilated veins, causing tightness and aching in the affected area. Blood does not flow smoothly through them, and a clot can form in the veins. Although many books advise one not to massage legs with varicose veins, I find that very gentle massage can be of tremendous benefit and can relieve the aching caused by this condition.

Do, however, check with a doctor first. If he agrees, you can give a very gentle massage. I must stress that all your movements should be extremely slow, gentle and soothing. Stroke round the varicose vein, but never massage on the vein itself as you could dislodge a clot, which can have serious, even fatal, consequences. So if the vein is particularly swollen or hard, be especially careful. Avoid all stimulating movements such as pummelling and hacking.

MASSAGE TECHNIQUE

This massage has a remarkably soothing effect on the legs, making them feel lighter and much more comfortable. You can do it to someone else, or massage your own legs. If you are massaging yourself, put your legs up: it is probably easiest to sit on the floor and rest your feet on a low stool.

1 Gently stroke the area around the vein. Stroke up the leg, working on either side of any visible veins.

2 Stroke the whole thigh from the knee upwards.

3 Stroke round the kneecap with your thumbs, then stroke behind your knee with your fingers, stroking gently up the leg.

4 Stroke up the calf, being careful not to press on any visible veins.

RHEUMATISM AND ARTHRITIS

The term rheumatism is used to describe any painful condition of the main structures of the body: the muscles, bones, joints, ligaments or tendons. Arthritis is a form of rheumatism in which the joints are affected. There are about 25 different types of arthritis, the two most common being osteoarthritis and rheumatoid arthritis. Massage can reduce the pain of both these disorders, but unfortunately it cannot cure the problem. Never do passive movements on an arthritic joint or massage directly on an inflamed or swollen joint.

OSTEOARTHRITIS

This name is given to the general wear and tear of joints associated with ageing. As we grow older, the cartilage degenerates, the ends of our bones become roughened and our joints are less well lubricated, resulting in stiffness and pain. Osteoarthritis usually affects the major weight-bearing joints, such as hips and knees, or joints that were injured earlier in life. It is made worse by any strain on the joint, and by being overweight.

Gentle massage can soothe the pain by warming and comforting the whole area. Pain from osteoarthritis is often caused not just by the joint itself, but by the surrounding muscles, which react to a damaged joint by going into spasm. Massage in warm water is also extremely comforting, as one of my clients, who had osteoarthritis in her knees, wrote to tell me: "I get into a fairly warm bath, to which I add one tablespoon of salt, and proceed to massage my thighs gently. I work from the thighs to the knees, and then, with both hands, softly explore the knee area (which is the most painful). I rub and apply slight pressure to the area where it hurts most. Then I lie back in the bath and relax, and in a short time the pain is gone."

RHEUMATOID ARTHRITIS

This is a condition in which the joints become inflamed, swollen and extremely painful. It usually affects the small joints of the hands and feet first, gradually spreading to other joints in the body.

Massage above and below the swollen area can help to relieve pain by relaxing the muscles and stimulating the lymphatic system. This speeds up the removal of waste products, thus reducing the swelling. Never massage directly on the swelling. If you are working on the hands or feet, stroke gently up the limb towards the lymph nodes in the armpit or groin (see manual lymph drainage, page 126).

Giving a massage

Use any of the techniques in the basic hand or foot massage (see pages 38 to 41 and 50 to 53) that your friend finds comforting. The movements below are particularly useful on arthritic joints in the hands.

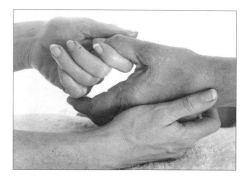

1 Stroke gently all around the joint, then do very light circular pressures on the joint with your thumb.

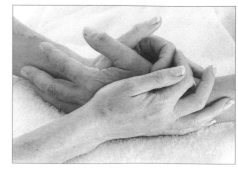

2 Gently stroke the whole hand to soothe it.

BACKACHE

Eight out of ten people in industrialized countries suffer from back pain at some time in their lives. Young or old, office workers or sportsmen, few of us escape the occasional backache. While it may be no more than a twinge, back pain can be extremely painful, rather frightening and, if the pain is constant, utterly exhausting. Yet a great deal of this trouble could be avoided if we looked after our backs better. We abuse them by standing badly or slouching over desks. We either do no exercise at all, or suddenly overdo it – and then wonder why we have backache. If we did regular exercise to keep our back and abdomen muscles strong and flexible, a lot of backache could be avoided.

Back pain is not just a physical problem: it is closely linked to mental stress and can be a physical manifestation of anxiety. It is more than a co-incidence that people with emotional problems – such as going through a divorce or being made redundant – often develop back pain. With its ability to reduce stress, massage can prevent or alleviate backache.

About 80 to 90 per cent of backache is caused by painful muscles. Massage is an ideal therapy for releasing minor muscular spasms and easing tense or strained muscles. However, if the pain is caused by damage to the spine, massage could worsen the condition, so do not use it unless you are sure that the pain is muscular. If your friend has pain running down an arm or a leg, refer him to a doctor or osteopath. Shiatsu may be helpful if your friend has sciatica.

GIVING A MASSAGE

Provided the backache is not very severe and that it is caused by aching muscles, you can massage the painful area gently. It is particularly important to make sure that your friend is lying comfortably, so use plenty of cushions as extra padding.

The treatment depends on your friend's preferences – you must respond to his needs. I usually begin by gently massaging the area surrounding the most painful part, trying to release any spasm in the muscles, and then apply slow, deep pressures to the tender spots. Use lots of smooth, rhythmic stroking movements, and avoid all pummelling and hacking. Deep, slow kneading can be very relaxing, but if the muscles are badly strained it may be too painful. Never do anything that hurts your friend, since this will make the muscles tighten up.

If the pain is very severe, or if the doctor does not advise back massage, you can still help your friend by massaging some other area of the body. This will help him to relax and feel more comfortable, which will speed his recovery from back pain. Try massaging the reflex area of the feet (see Reflexology, pages 120 to 124), or work gently on the abdomen.

SHIATSU

Sciatic pain can be eased by pressing with your thumbs on certain shiatsu points. Apply the pressure with care, since these points may be very tender, hold for about ten seconds, then move on to the next point.

1 *Press on either side of the spine at the small of the back (Bladder 26).*

2 *Press at the back of the thighs directly under the buttocks (Bladder 36).*

3 *Press in the middle of the back of the thighs (Bladder 37).*

4 *Press in the centre of the hollow on the side of the buttocks (Gall bladder 30).*

5 *Press half way down the side of the thigh (Gall bladder 31).*

6 *Press half way down the back of the calf (Bladder 57).*

CANCER

I first became interested in massaging cancer patients when a friend's mother was dying of cancer. She felt isolated, frightened and anxious, and massage was able to calm her down almost miraculously. She had a nurse who felt powerless to help her, and who just sat reading in the next room, thoroughly bored. Had the nurse been able to massage her patient, both of them would have benefited. The dying woman would have felt comforted, her tension and anxiety would have been relieved. The nurse would have felt happier at being able to give some positive help. It was this situation that made me decide to work in the British National Health Service and teach nurses how to massage so that everyone could benefit.

People who are really ill often feel very isolated and lonely. A massage can make all the difference in the world. There are no special techniques for massaging cancer patients: any massage is comforting. Touch is a way of expressing concern and sympathy, and induces warmth and relaxation, which can help to ease pain.

DRUG REHABILITATION

Anyone who is trying to come off drugs will benefit from a regular massage. Drug addicts often suffer from a tremendous sense of shame: they know they have disappointed everyone, they feel ostracized and untouchable. The fact that someone is prepared to give them some attention and to touch them helps them regain both their self-esteem and their desire to get well. For once their bodies, which they have so abused, are receiving attention and they realize that there are other ways of feeling good apart from taking drugs. As one girl said, "I didn't think it was possible to feel high without drugs." By relaxing and experiencing a new form of pleasure, drug addicts are able to remember their pre-drug days, and regain respect for their bodies. The mother of one addict said that having a massage was the turning point in her daughter's recovery.

Drug addicts tend to lead unhealthy lives. Their circulation is bad and they suffer from cold extremities. Massage improves the circulation and makes the body feel more alive.

Heroin is a total muscle relaxant and nerve sedative. When an addict withdraws, he loses the ability to relax, and so becomes extremely tense. One ex-addict said, "I felt terrible when I was withdrawing, and didn't think anything apart from heroin would help. I was delighted to find that after having a full body massage my body felt totally at ease. The shivering stopped as I felt warmer. My muscles stopped cramping and my nerves weren't jumping around so much. I also felt much less depressed and for a few minutes the world didn't seem so awful." She found massage so beneficial that she decided to learn how to massage, so that she could help other people in the same situation. She came to my courses and found that being able to help someone else greatly improved her self-esteem.

SLIMMING

Whenever massage and slimming are mentioned together, a cynic is bound to say that massage is of no use, and that the only one to lose weight is the masseur. This is not true. Massage can help you to slim. Although it does not break down fat, and so alone cannot reduce weight, it can improve your self-image and appearance, and that will help you to slim. Massage gives you a positive image of your own body, which reminds you to hold yourself better and stand straighter. That alone will make you look better. Many slimmers have a distorted image of their bodies: they imagine themselves to be much larger and fatter than they really are. Massage can help to give you an indication of your true size.

As the treatment helps you to feel better and take a pride in your body, it means that you are more likely to keep to a diet, and so your chances of losing weight are greatly enhanced. The knowledge that the person giving the massage is going to look critically at your body, and will notice whether you have lost a pound or two, will also encourage you to keep to a diet.

Added to this are other benefits to the appearance. By stimulating the circulation, massage tones the skin and smoothes the body. This improvement builds a positive self-image, which produces energy, making exercising easier. The upwards spiral has begun, and weight will come off more easily.

MASSAGE TECHNIQUES

If you are helping a slimmer to lose weight, follow the general sequence given in Chapter 1. Spend more time on the fleshiest areas, particularly the abdomen, thighs and buttocks, and do plenty of stimulating movements such as kneading and pummelling.

The abdomen and thighs are easy to massage yourself, and you can help your weight-watching programme with a few minutes of vigorous massage each day.

1 Lie on your back and knead your abdomen thoroughly, doing several rows of kneading across it to cover the whole area.

2 Roll onto one side, then knead and pummel your hip. Repeat on the other side.

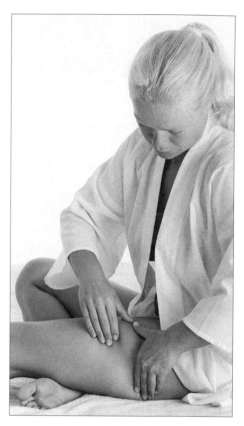

3 Sit up and knead your thighs from the knee up to the top. Work vigorously on the front and outside, but more gently on the inside.

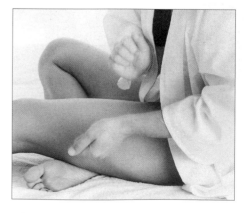

4 Pummel very fast all over the front and outside of your thighs, then work more gently on the inside.

SHIATSU

Press these points firmly for seven to ten seconds each. They help weight-loss by suppressing the appetite and stimulating the metabolism.

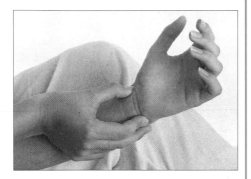

1 Squeeze either side of the wrist above the wrist bones (Heart 7).

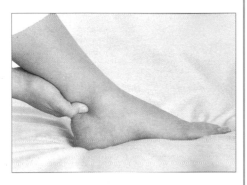

2 Press on the inside edge of the ankle, in the hollow just behind the bony prominence (Kidney 3).

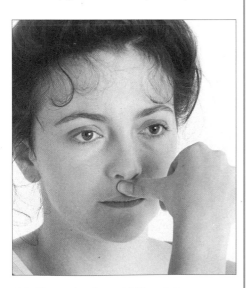

3 Press in the middle of the groove running from the nose to the upper lip (Governing vessel 26).

SHIATSU QUICK CURES

Although shiatsu is really a treatment for toning up the whole body (see pages 114 to 119), there are several very useful points that can provide quick remedies for minor ailments.

Press on the relevant points for between three and seven seconds. Bear in mind that you are treating the symptoms, not the cause of your health problem. If the cure lasts only a short time and the disorder keeps returning, you should consult a doctor or have a complete shiatsu treatment done by a professional.

COMMON COLD

1 *On the web of skin between the thumb and forefinger (Large intestine 4).*

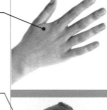

2 *On the indentations at the base of the skull (Governing vessel 15 and Gall bladder 20).*

3 *At the base of the neck, on either side of the vertebrae, and about three finger widths below (Bladder 12 and 13).*

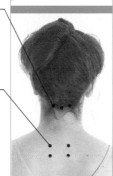

STOMACH ACHE

1 *Three finger widths below the navel (Conception vessel 6).*

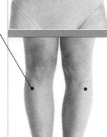

2 *In the groove behind the shin bone, four finger widths below the knee (Stomach 36).*

MENSTRUAL PAIN

Squeeze on either side of the ankle just behind the bony prominence, and on the inside of the leg about four finger widths above the prominence (Kidney 3, Bladder 60 and Spleen 6).

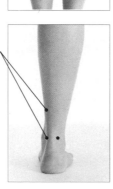

ACHING LEGS

In the groove behind the shin bone, four finger widths below the knee (Stomach 36).

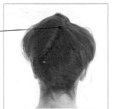

HANGOVER

Crown of the head (Governing vessel 20).

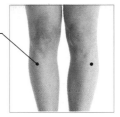

TOOTHACHE

On the web of skin between the thumb and forefinger (Large intestine 4).

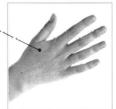

LACK OF ENERGY

1 *Just below the ball of the foot in the centre of the sole (Kidney 1). This point has the apt name of "gushing spring".*

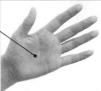

2 *Squeeze the middle of the palm of the hand (Heart constrictor 8).*

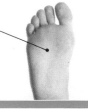

3 *In the groove behind the shin bone, four finger widths below the knee (Stomach 36).*

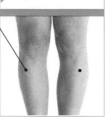

EXERCISE

Sportsmen and women have always known of the value of massage. It is the perfect adjunct to exercise: it restores muscular power and mobility, and can banish muscular spasms. It also stimulates the lymphatic flow, thus assisting in the removal of waste products which accumulate during exercise. As the Greek physician, Hippocrates, noted in the third century BC, massage can ease stiff joints. "The physician must be experienced in many things, but assuredly also in rubbing . . . for rubbing can bind a joint that is too loose and loosen a joint that is too hard."

Massage can complement and enhance your exercise programme. You can use it before exercise to warm up and loosen the body, or after exercise to help prevent stiff muscles and a build-up of waste products. It can also relieve cramps and speed up recovery from sprained joints. Massage maintains muscles at the peak of their flexibility and strength, so that you can perform at your best.

In my practice the runners, ballerinas and cyclists that we treat all claim that after a massage their minds are clear and relaxed, and their performances are greatly improved. A marathon runner felt he could run for ever; a sprinter felt he had more power; a cyclist finds it keeps his legs fit, and several ballerinas would not be without it, since they are so much more supple afterwards.

I have also experienced the benefits of massage after strenuous exercise. While on a trip to Sarawak, I was fortunate enough to make an excursion to the Niah caves. To reach the massive caves we had to walk three kilometres through the jungle on a plank walk. We then spent several hours exploring before walking back down. I thought my legs would be agony the next day, so I had a massage that evening.

A small elderly lady came; she was the local midwife and told me she had delivered at least 1,000 babies. The massage was done on the floor, one brightly-coloured sarong underneath me and another one on top. She massaged with coconut oil in which she had soaked a mixture of herbs and spices including peppercorns, anise, cardamom and turmeric. On places that were particularly painful, she used an oil into which she had crushed a small red onion. Her smallness belied her strength, and when she did my legs I thought I would scream – but the next day I could have happily repeated the trek.

PRE-EXERCISE MASSAGE

If your muscles are tense before you start exercising, your performance will be badly affected. Muscles work in pairs, one contracting as the other relaxes. If one of the pair is tense, the other has to work harder than usual, since it is working against the resistance of the tense, shortened muscle. Simply by being tense, the muscles are doing more work than is necessary, giving off more wastes and using up more oxygen.

Ideally, do a whole body massage. Most sports put a demand on the legs, buttocks and back muscles, so massage these areas very thoroughly. If you do not have time for this, massage the muscles your friend will be using, concentrating on any areas of tension. Use a lot of fast kneading movements, and instead of finishing your massage with soporific stroking, use a stimulating movement such as pummelling to increase blood supply.

MASSAGE AFTER EXERCISE

Nearly 1,000 years ago, Avicenna, one of the greatest physicians and philosophers of his time, wrote: "As a sequel to athletics, restorative friction produces repose. Its object is to dispense the effete matters formed in the muscles and not expelled by exercise. It causes them to disperse and so removes fatigue and the feeling of lassitude."

During exercise, waste products such as lactic and carbolic acids and urea are released into the muscles. It is

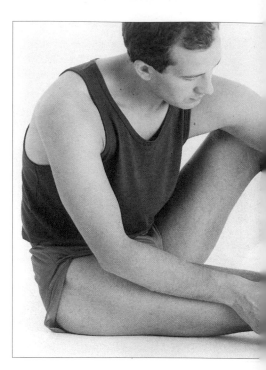

the accumulation of these wastes that can cause stiffness and pain. The lymphatic system drains them out of the body, but this can take several hours or even a few days. Massage, with its pumping and stroking action, can speed up their elimination.

It is essential to keep the muscles warm after exercise, so make sure that the room is well heated. If you have time, massage the entire body, paying more attention to those areas stressed by the exercise. Massage firmly towards the heart at the beginning of the massage, but finish each section with very gentle stroking towards the lymph nodes (see manual lymph drainage, page 126). If there is any sign of injury, avoid that area until you have consulted a doctor.

CUTS AND BRUISES

Minor injuries can be soothed with massage, which stimulates the healing process. Never massage directly on an injury, just work very gently around it, stroking towards the nearest lymph nodes, and kneading very gently above and to the side of the injury. When massaging around any injury, ask your friend to tell you if there is any tenderness or discomfort, and if so, work further away from the injury.

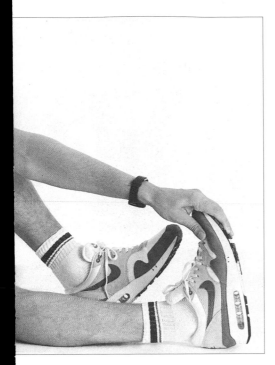

Do not massage around an open wound, or on a bruised area unless you know the cause of the bruising. Bruises developing without an obvious cause can be a symptom of serious illness, so your friend should consult a doctor.

CRAMPS

If you are prone to cramps during or after exercise, massage will definitely help. A cramped muscle is tightly contracted and the blood supply is reduced. Massage stretches the muscle and improves circulation, leaving it more flexible.

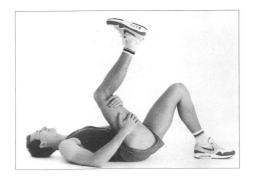

HAMSTRING CRAMP: *Lie on your back and raise the affected leg. Stroke the back of your thigh firmly, then knead it. Finally, stroke the area again to soothe it.*

CALF CRAMPS: ◀ *Sit with the affected leg straight, and bend your foot up so that you stretch the calf muscle. Then knead the muscle firmly, working up your leg. When you feel the muscle relaxing, soothe it by rhythmically stroking down the whole leg.*

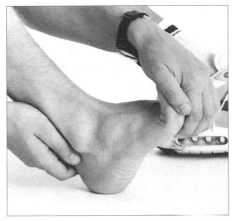

FOOT CRAMP: *Grasp your toes, and gently but firmly bend them back while holding your heel with your other hand. Stroke and knead the sole of the foot.*

STRAINS AND SPRAINS

A strain is simply overstretching of the muscles and involves no swelling, whereas a sprain is an abnormal wrenching or twisting of the joint. In a sprain there may be damage to the associated ligaments, tendons, muscles, blood vessels or nerves. A severely sprained joint is extremely painful and swollen, and cannot be moved. Gentle massage can accelerate healing for both strains and sprains.

Apply a cold compress to the area as soon as possible – a packet of frozen peas is ideal. Leave this on for about 15 minutes. If the joint is extremely painful, consult a doctor because there could be a fracture. If you think there is no fracture, you can massage very gently around the injury after removing the cold compress.

Start by stroking gently above the site of the injury, working towards the nearest lymph nodes. This will help to drain away the accumulation of blood and fluids around the injury, which are the main cause of swelling.

Sprained ankle

The most common place for a sprain is the ankle. Very gentle massage can help to reduce swelling and relieve pain. Ask your friend to tell you if the massage is painful: if it is, work further away from the injury. Massage for at least ten minutes, and repeat several times a day. Continue this treatment regularly for about a week or until the injury is healed.

1 Start by gently stroking up the thigh towards the lymph nodes in the groin.

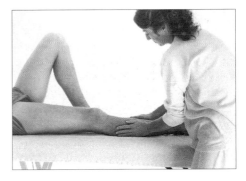

2 Stroke up the sides of the calf to the knee and glide gently back down to the ankle.

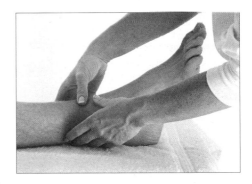

3 Stroke extremely gently with short upwards movements all round the ankle using your thumbs.

Other sprained joints

A sprained wrist can be treated in much the same way, stroking gently towards the lymph nodes in the armpits and the elbow. However, a sprained knee should always be examined by a doctor: do not attempt to massage it without first obtaining a doctor's consent.

ANATOMY

In order to give someone an effective, relaxing massage, it is useful to know something about the structure beneath your hands: where the bones are and what lies under them; where the muscles are, whether they are large or small, and what they do. The working of the body is fascinating: it is a miraculous machine which few of us really appreciate. As you give a massage, you will probably find yourself wanting to know more about how it functions. A basic knowledge of anatomy will give you the confidence to judge when or where a massage will be most beneficial, and help you to understand the value of massage.

MUSCLES

In massage you are working primarily on the muscular system, which makes up about 40 per cent of our body weight. All movements of the body are brought about by the contraction of muscles. These are bundles of extremely elastic fibres that respond to signals from the brain. There are two types of muscles in the body. Those under conscious control are called voluntary muscles: the muscles in your limbs, for example, move your arms and legs when you decide to move. Other muscles, known as involuntary muscles, are not under conscious control. Involuntary muscles include the heart muscle and the muscles of the digestive system.

When muscles contract, they need oxygen and glucose to provide energy. They give off waste products, including lactic acid, carbon dioxide and urea, after a period of activity. These waste products are drained from the area by the blood circulation and through the lymph system (see page 141), but if too much accumulates, the muscles can feel tired, stiff and painful. Excess lactic acid may cause cramps. Massage can help the recovery of stiff, painful or over-tired muscles by speeding up the elimination of waste products and temporarily increasing the local blood supply.

SKELETON

Composed of some 206 separate bones, the skeleton provides the framework for the body, giving it strength and shape. Vital organs, such as the brain, spinal cord, heart and lungs are encased in bony structures to protect them from damage. Muscles and tendons are attached to bones, allowing movement of all parts of the body.

The male and female skeletons differ only slightly: the male skeleton is generally larger and heavier, while the female has a wider pelvis.

BONES

These are the hardest of all living tissue, and store calcium and phosphorus. Some have a soft inner core, the bone marrow, which is responsible for manufacturing most of the blood cells. Bones vary in size and shape, from the long ones in the limbs – the largest of all being the femur in the thigh – to tiny ones in the fingers, toes and the cavities of the middle ear.

HOW MUSCLES WORK

Most voluntary muscles are attached with tendons to a bone at either end, straddling a joint. They are generally arranged in pairs, one on either side of the bone. When one muscle contracts, it pulls the bone towards it, and the muscle on the other side relaxes to accommodate the movement.

RELAXED MUSCLE

CONTRACTED MUSCLE

TENDON

BONE

JOINTS

There are several types of joint allowing a different range of movement combined with varying degrees of strength. Certain joints, such as those between the bones making up the skull, are immovable. In a movable joint, the ends of the bones are covered in smooth cartilage. A capsule round the joint exudes a thick, viscous fluid to lubricate it. A casing of strong, flexible fibres called ligaments, binds the joint firmly together.

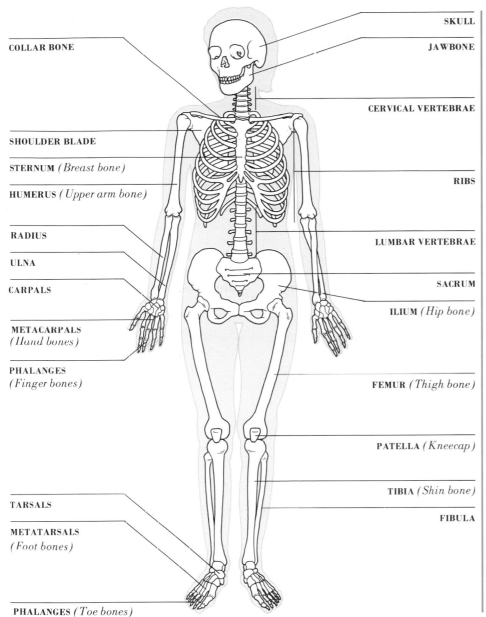

COLLAR BONE

SHOULDER BLADE

STERNUM (Breast bone)

HUMERUS (Upper arm bone)

RADIUS

ULNA

CARPALS

METACARPALS
(Hand bones)

PHALANGES
(Finger bones)

TARSALS

METATARSALS
(Foot bones)

PHALANGES (Toe bones)

SKULL

JAWBONE

CERVICAL VERTEBRAE

RIBS

LUMBAR VERTEBRAE

SACRUM

ILIUM (Hip bone)

FEMUR (Thigh bone)

PATELLA (Kneecap)

TIBIA (Shin bone)

FIBULA

SKIN

For the purpose of massage, the most important organ is the skin. It is the largest organ of the body, that of an adult man weighing about 3kg (6lbs). An elastic, waterproof covering, it acts as a barrier against infection and regulates body temperature.

The skin is made up of two layers. The outer layer (the epidermis) is a mass of cells in two levels. The uppermost level is composed of dead cells which flake away all the time. Beneath this are living cells which grow outwards gradually.

The underlying layer, the dermis, is a jelly-like substance containing blood and lymph vessels, sebaceous and sweat glands, hair follicles and nerve endings. Some areas of the body, such as the fingertips and lips, have millions of nerve endings and are extremely sensitive. Other areas, such as the back, have far fewer nerve endings and are much less sensitive.

The skin has an ample supply of blood to nourish it and to allow the replacement of cells as they die off. By improving the circulation, massage helps to maintain healthy cells and so imparts a healthy glow to the skin. Indeed, the health of the skin is a very accurate reflection of the state of the whole body. It has been called the "external nervous system", and the Chinese refer to it as "the third lung".

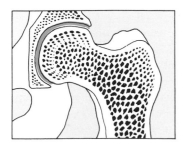

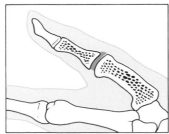

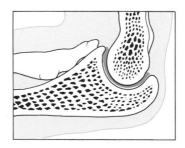

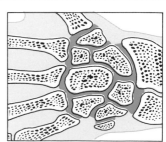

BALL AND SOCKET JOINTS, *such as the hips (above) and shoulders, allow maximum range of movement, combined with great strength.*

SADDLE JOINTS *at the thumbs also allow free movement in all directions, but are not as strong as ball and socket joints.*

HINGE JOINTS *allow movement in one direction only. Examples are the knees and finger joints and the elbows, illustrated above.*

GLIDING JOINTS, *such as the wrists, allow movement in all directions, but they are more restricted than saddle joints.*

HEART AND CIRCULATION

The cardio-vascular system comprises the heart, blood and the vessels that carry the blood. As well as regulating body temperature, it has the vital roles of transporting and distributing nutrients and oxygen to the billions of cells in the body and removing any waste products which those cells may have produced. These supplies allow the whole body – muscles, skin, bones and internal organs – to grow, repair damage and carry out their various functions. Massage improves the blood circulation without putting any extra strain on the heart. Thus it increases the supply of oxygen and nutrients to local areas.

Blood is pumped from the heart through a complex system of blood vessels to the entire body. The vessels that carry blood away from the heart, called arteries, branch out into smaller and smaller ones, the smallest of which, called capillaries, form a network throughout the body. The walls of capillaries are very thin, so that nutrients and oxygen in the blood can pass through them to the surrounding tissue, and carbon dioxide, which is produced as a waste product, passes from the tissues into the blood. These tiny blood vessels then join up into larger ones, finally into large veins which carry blood back to the right side of the heart and from there to the lungs.

At every heart beat, blood is pumped out at high pressure, and it is these waves of pressure that you can feel at pulse points. Arteries have strong, elastic walls to withstand the changes in pressure within them.

Blood is at a much lower pressure in the veins, and they have much thinner, less elastic walls. At intervals along the veins there are valves which prevent the blood flowing backwards. If these valves are damaged, allowing blood to flow backwards, varicose veins may result.

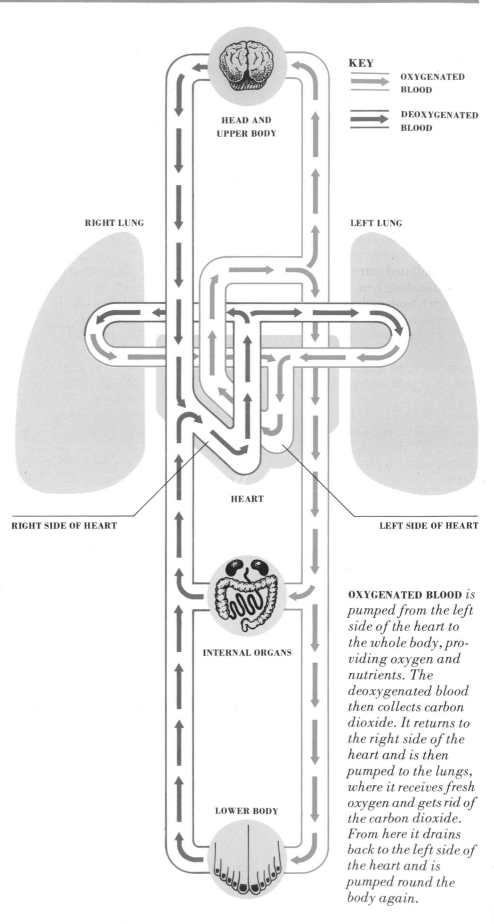

KEY

→ OXYGENATED BLOOD

➤ DEOXYGENATED BLOOD

HEAD AND UPPER BODY

RIGHT LUNG

LEFT LUNG

HEART

RIGHT SIDE OF HEART

LEFT SIDE OF HEART

INTERNAL ORGANS

LOWER BODY

OXYGENATED BLOOD *is pumped from the left side of the heart to the whole body, providing oxygen and nutrients. The deoxygenated blood then collects carbon dioxide. It returns to the right side of the heart and is then pumped to the lungs, where it receives fresh oxygen and gets rid of the carbon dioxide. From here it drains back to the left side of the heart and is pumped round the body again.*

THE LYMPHATIC SYSTEM

All cells of the body are bathed in a fluid known as extracellular fluid. The lymphatic system purifies this fluid and ensures that the cells have a healthy environment to live in. It is via the extracellular fluid that nutrients and waste products pass between the blood and the cells. Some waste products cannot pass directly back into the blood, and begin to accumulate in the extracellular fluid.

The polluted extracellular fluid circulates along lymph vessels and through lymph nodes (also called lymph glands), which filter out waste products and bacteria. The vessels link up, becoming larger and larger in much the same way as blood vessels, and eventually drain back into the veins. When it is in the lymph vessels, extracellular fluid is known as lymph.

There are lymph vessels and nodes throughout the body. The nodes are in the neck, armpits, groin, behind the knees and on the inside of the elbows. The spleen, thymus and tonsils are also part of this system.

The lymphatic system plays an important part in fighting infection and developing immunity to disease. Lymph nodes and the lymphatic organs such as the thymus manufacture lymphocytes, a type of white blood cell which fights infection. The nodes also act as filters to prevent the spread of infection through the body, and since they help to block the infection, it is common for them to become swollen and painful during illness. Unlike the blood circulation, the lymphatic system has no heart to pump lymph through the body. Its movement is dependent on muscular contraction and aided by valves in the lymph vessels. Consequently, pressure in the lymph vessels is low, and lymphatic drainage is easily restricted. Massage can help in pumping the lymph through the body, thus eliminating waste and strengthening the immune system.

THE NERVOUS SYSTEM

The most complex system of the body, the nervous system has the vital role of regulating the many and varied activities of the body, and relaying messages from all parts of the body to the brain, and from the brain back again. Nerves leave the brain at the base of the skull, and extend down the back in a rope-like bunch called the spinal cord. They are protected by the vertebrae of the spine, which form a bony channel. Massage affects the nervous system, and can have either a sedative or a stimulating effect.

SENSORY AND MOTOR NERVES

The nerves that collect information and relay it to the brain are known as sensory nerves, those that carry messages from the brain to the muscles and glands are known as motor nerves.

There are millions of sensory nerve endings, or receptors, throughout the body, each specialized to respond to different types of stimuli. Whilst the receptors in the eyes and ears are sensitive to light and sound waves, different receptors in the skin respond to pain, pressure and heat. There are receptors in the joints, muscles and tendons, relaying information about the position of limbs. All these nerves carry information up the spinal cord to the brain in the form of electrical impulses. The brain processes the information, and if it decides to take action, messages are relayed through the motor nerves to the appropriate muscles or glands.

Reflex actions may be initiated in the spinal cord instead of the brain. If you burn your finger, for instance, the pain message is processed in the spinal cord, and the reflex action of pulling your hand away from the hot surface is initiated immediately, before the pain message has reached the brain.

AUTONOMIC NERVOUS SYSTEM

There are also receptors to pick up information about blood pressure, acidity levels in the stomach, the level of carbon dioxide in the blood and so on. This information is dealt with subconsciously, and appropriate changes in heart beat or secretion of digestive juices are initiated by the brain. The part of the nervous system that regulates functions not under our conscious control is known as the autonomic nervous system.

SECTION THROUGH THE SPINE

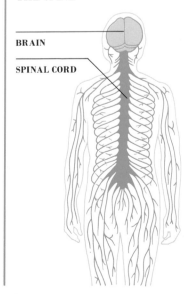

BRAIN

SPINAL CORD

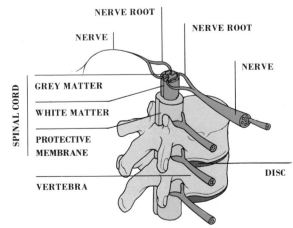

SPINAL CORD

NERVE ROOT

NERVE

NERVE ROOT

NERVE

GREY MATTER

WHITE MATTER

PROTECTIVE MEMBRANE

VERTEBRA

DISC

PAIRS OF NERVES *emerge through gaps between each pair of adjacent vertebrae, and branch out to reach the entire body.*

INDEX

BIBLIOGRAPHY

Beard, G. and Wood, E. *Massage – Principles and Techniques*. Saunders, 1964.

Benson, H M O. *Relaxation Response*. Fontana, 1977.

Cyriax, J M O. *Treatment by Massage and Manipulation*. 1948.

Delvin, Dr D. *You and Your Back*. Pan, 1975.

Downing, G. *The Massage Book*. Wildwood House, 1973.

Graham, D M O. *Massage, Manual Treatment and Remedial Movements*. 1913.

Groddeck, G. *The Meaning of Illness*. Hogarth Press, 1977.

Hearn, Editha. *You are as Young as your Spine*. Heinemann, 1975.

Hinrichsen. *The Body Book*. Taplinger, 1967.

Inkeles, G. *The Art of Sensual Massage*. George, Allen and Unwin, 1973.

Inkeles, G. *The New Massage*. George, Allen and Unwin, 1980.

Johnson, W, MD. *The Anatriptic Art*. 1866.

Krieger, Dolores. *Therapeutic Touch*. Prentice Hall, 1979.

Lauder Brunton, Sir T, MD. *Circulation and Respiration*. 1907.

Leboyer, Frederick. *Loving Hands*. Knopf, 1976.

Lettvin, Maggie. *The Back Book*. Houghton Mifflin Co, 1976.

Liddell, Lucy. *The Book of Massage*. Ebury Press, 1984.

Mackenzie, Sir James. *Diseases of the Heart*. 1908.

Madders, Jane. *Stress and Relaxation*. Martin Dunitz, 1979.

McGuinan, J. *Stress and Tension Control*. Plenum Press, 1980.

Mennel, J B. *Physical Treatment by Movement and Massage*. Churchill Ltd, 1917.

Mitchel, Laura. *Simple Relaxation*. John Murray, 1977.

Mitchel, Laura and Dale, Barbara. *Simple Movement*. John Murray, 1980.

Montague, Ashley. *Touching*. Columbia Press, 1971.

Morrison, A, MD. FRCP. *Cardiac Failure*. 1897.

Murrell, W, MD. FRCP. *Massotherapeutics or Massage as a Mode of Treatment*. 1886.

Ornstein, R. *The Amazing Brain*. Chatto and Windus, 1986.

Prudden, Bonnie. *Pain Erasure*. Ballantine, 1980.

Rayner, Dr. *Practical Remarks on Treatment of Various Diseases by Manipulation*. 1862.

Simonton, Carl and Stephanie. *Getting Well Again*. Bantam, 1986.

Vincent, L M, MD. *The Dancers' Book of Health*. Sheed Andrews and McMeal Inc, 1978.

Emotional Deprivation in Infants. Journal of Pediatrics, Vol 35, 1949.

PHYSIOLOGY
McMinn, R M H and Hutchings, R T. *A Colour Atlas of Human Anatomy*. Wolfe Medical Publications.

SHIATSU
Antri Medical School Hospital. *Chinese Massage Therapy*. Routledge and Kegan Paul, 1983.

Beresford-Cooke, Carola. *The Book of Massage* (shiatsu section). Ebury Press, 1984.

Chan, Pedro. *Finger Acupressure*. Ballantine, 1974.

Kurland, Howard, MD. *Quick Headache Relief*.

Namikoshi, Tokujiro. *Shiatsu*. Japan Publications, 1972.

Namikoshi, Toru. *Complete Shiatsu Therapy*. Japan Publications, 1981.

Ohashi, Wataru. *Do-it-Yourself Shiatsu*. Duttons, 1976.

Prudden, Bonnie. *Myotherapy*. Ballantine, 1984.

Yamomoto, Shikuku. *Barefoot Shiatsu*. Japan Publications, 1979.

REFLEXOLOGY
Bayley, Doreen. *Reflexology Today*. Doreen Bayley, 1978.

Byers, Dwight. *Better Health with Foot Reflexology*. Ingham Publishing Inc, 1983.

Kunz, Kevin and Barbara. *The Complete Guide to Foot Reflexology*. Prentice Hall, 1982.

ACKNOWLEDGMENTS

AUTHOR'S ACKNOWLEDGMENTS
I would like to thank the following people: Carola Beresford-Cooke for her help with the shiatsu section; Pan Wade for her help on the reflexology section; Philip Beach and Tony Llycholat for their help with the anatomy and physiology; Daphne Van Renen for the original editing; Helena Edwards for deciphering my writing and typing the original manuscript; Anne Vadgama, Gill Whitworth, Jo Jones, Amina Shah and Jenny Gilroy for their help and encouragement; Dr Peter Nixon, Dr David Sobel and Professor R. Ornstein; my clients, patients and students for all that they have taught me over the years; everyone at Dorling Kindersley, especially Mark for all his painstaking care and Claire for editing; finally I want to thank Sandra Lousada for her beautiful photographs.

DORLING KINDERSLEY would like to thank: Joanna Martin for her help with art direction; Hannah Moore for her design assistance; Richard and Hilary Bird for the index; G. Baldwin and Co for the vegetable oils (pages 18-19); Hilary Guy; Fanny Rush; The Futon Company; Futon Furnishing; and all our models – Winni Olesen, Paul Johnson, Frances Graham, Martha Fraton and Paul Surety from Pineapple Studios, Eve Tomlinson, Fran, Edward and Jake Tise, Tom and Hossein Razazan, Olivia Flecha, Jack Richards, India and Julia Balmforth, Susan Moore, Amina Shah, Tony Llycholat and Bob Gates.

MAKE-UP
Barbara Jones

ILLUSTRATORS
John Woodcock, Brian Sayers

TYPESETTING
Chambers Wallace, London
Airedale Graphics

REPRODUCTION
Reprocolor Llovet Barcelona SA

MASSAGE COURSES
For information on Clare Maxwell-Hudson's massage courses, write to PO Box 457, London NW2 4BR.

40/475/1